Beyond Diet © 2014 by Isabel De Los Rios

First edition published 2007
Second edition published 2008
Third edition published 2009
First hard-copy edition published 2010
Second hard-copy edition published 2010
Third hard-copy edition published 2011
Fourth hard-copy edition published 2011
Fifth hard-copy edition published 2012
Sixth hard-copy edition published 2014

Disclaimer

This manual is not intended to provide medical advice or to take the place of medical advice and treatment from your personal physician. Readers are advised to consult their own doctors or other qualified health professionals regarding the treatment of medical conditions. The author shall not be held liable or responsible for any misunderstanding or misuse of the information contained in this manual or for any loss, damage, or injury caused or alleged to be caused directly or indirectly by any treatment, action, or application of any food or food source discussed in this manual. The statements in this book have not been evaluated by the U.S. Food and Drug Administration. This information is not intended to diagnose, treat, cure, or prevent any disease.

To request permission for reproduction or inquire about private nutritional consulting or speaking engagements, contact:

Isabel De Los Rios
Live Smart Solutions
3452 Richville RD #1447
Manchester Center, VT 05255
E-mail: questions@beyonddiet.com

Contents

Preface

Does the world need another diet book? When I asked myself this question, I knew the answer clearly: No. People don't need another diet book; they need to change their lifestyles. They don't need to be told how and why to go on a diet; they need to learn how to change their eating habits and their thinking for life.

With all the diet books out there, why are so many Americans still overweight and in poor health? Unfortunately, the media bombards us with so much information daily that most people don't know what to believe. I've often heard from clients, "I just don't know what to eat anymore."

With this manual, my goal is to clarify what true nutrition is and which foods you should eat—not only to achieve an ideal weight but also to avoid the conditions that are all too common in this country today, such as high cholesterol, diabetes, and heart disease.

Am I just another nutritionist putting out just another nutrition program? I assure you that I am not. My quest for answers about optimum nutrition began 15 years ago. Since then, I have made it my life's work to study everything I could possibly get my hands on related to nutrition, exercise, and optimum health and weight. This means that I've studied the good and the bad. This manual contains the best information that I've found, culled from some of the most respected doctors and nutritionists who share a similar passion for nutrition.

Like most Americans, I had tried every diet out there and had been unsuccessful in the long term. Only after I recognized and accepted the principles taught in this manual was I able to achieve the optimum weight and health that I enjoy today.

How I nourish my body affects all aspects of my life, as well as my outlook on it. How do I feel when I wake up in the morning? GREAT! How do I feel when I get up in front of a crowd and give a lecture? GREAT! How do I feel when my day doesn't go as planned and things get overwhelming and a bit rough? GREAT!

I know that feeling great has everything to do with how I take care of my body and my health—and you can feel great, too.

Acknowledgements

I thank so many people for making this manual possible:

- God—through whom all things are possible.

- Oscar De Los Rios—whose passion for his work and his life taught me that being passionate about my own work and life is the only way to truly live a happy life.

- Pilar De Los Rios—whose personal struggle with type 2 diabetes and kidney disease taught me more about health and nutrition than any book ever could.

- Every author mentioned in this manual, especially Paul Chek— you have dedicated your lives to studying, researching, and teaching the world what you know is the truth about optimum nutrition. Through your work, I have been able to learn, benefit from, and share this vital information. I am a grateful student forever.

A special thanks to my business partner, Jeff Siegel. His patience and hard work made it possible for this manual to be transformed from an idea to a reality.

PART 1

If you're reading this manual, chances are that you've decided to make serious changes in your health and eating habits. Maybe you have tried several diets and exercise programs, without success. Maybe you have yo-yo dieted for years and are tired of the ups and downs. Hopefully, you have decided to commit yourself to a new way of living. Whether this is the first time you have tried to change your eating and lifestyle or you've been working toward it for a while, remember that looking and feeling good requires hard work and dedication. I can assure you that the results will be well worth the effort.

Why have other programs failed you? First, if you're like many people, you temporarily altered what you were eating but didn't change your eating habits, and after you stopped dieting, you returned to the habits that had put on the excess weight in the first place. Second, most diet programs don't consider your overall health; they are just "controlled starvation." Starvation slows your metabolism, so after you stop dieting, you may gain back even more weight as a result. Third, since you were essentially starving yourself, you were most likely experiencing symptoms of starvation (fatigue, sluggishness, and hunger). Who can stay motivated about a diet that doesn't make you feel healthy?

I tell all of my clients that if you don't have your health, nothing else matters. If you feel terrible when you wake up in the morning, then your whole day takes on the same somber tone. Promise yourself that from this point forward, you will commit to doing what it takes to keep your body healthy so that you can live a long life and wake up each morning feeling and looking your best!

Beyond Diet is a way to change your eating habits for life. You will develop a new long-term eating strategy—not modify your diet temporarily—by creating the best meal plan to suit you. You'll eat healthy foods that you enjoy and discover great new foods, too. You'll feel so good, you won't want to go back to your old habits. From this day forward, you will be able to say, I'm committed to keeping myself healthy and happy.

Say it with me:

I'm committed to keeping myself healthy and happy.

And there will be no turning back.

All that said, I want you to know that my own healthy transition did not happen overnight. It took me three years before I was able to implement every principle I am going to teach you in this program. Three years is a long time, and I suspect you can make it happen faster than I did. Much of that time was spent searching and researching the best and most up to date nutrition information so I could put it into a manual for your benefit. Would it have been ideal for me to transform every aspect of my diet overnight? Sure, that would have been great. However, that was not realistic for me at the time and it may not be for you either. I am actually extremely grateful I implemented each healthy principle over a period of time. Making these changes slowly helped me to truly adopt these principles as a lifestyle and not as a temporary diet fix.

Many people assume they will have to "give up" all of their favorite foods to enjoy their ideal weight and good health. I am not asking you to give up anything! This is not a crash diet, it is a lifestyle change. Living the life you want to live may require you to focus more on certain healthy foods over others, but does not require you to give up every delicious food available. If you think I have given up some of my favorite foods like chocolate and wine, I assure you this is not the case. The difference is that now I know where these foods fit into my meal plan and how I can enjoy them while still maintaining my weight and feeling great.

The same goes for you. Don't throw in the towel or give up because you think you can't do every single principle, every single day. This is not an all or nothing deal. It is you implementing each principle the best you can, each and every day.

I encourage you to take charge of your health and your weight one step at a time. If you do what you can in the short term, these principles will become a permanent part of your lifestyle in the long term. Remember, I was where you are now or, quite possibly, in a much more challenging position. Hundreds of my clients were as well. One small change at a time and they have found a new sense of health and vitality that they did not think was possible for them. Not only are they now feeling great, but they are able to keep their weight off permanently, once and for all.

The steps required to achieve your ideal weight and health are exactly like those of any long term goal. Imagine you wanted to start your own business. Would you expect to be "Open for Business" overnight? Of course not; you would do your research, follow a plan, and take one step each day to bring you closer to success.

What do you need to do to achieve your weight loss and health goals? One thing that you can easily do is to keep asking yourself: "Is this choice I'm about to make bringing me closer to my goal or taking me further from it?" Choose which direction you want to go and commit yourself to making it happen.

People often regret the things they don't do, not the things they do. What will you regret if you don't take care of your health and weight today? Let's eliminate all possible regrets and make your dreams your reality.

1: A Program for Success

Achieving success in any weight-loss program takes more than just following nutritional information; it requires getting into the right state of mind. All of our actions are governed by our thoughts. If it is true that thoughts create reality, then it is imperative to create the environment that will support a successful meal plan.

In this chapter, I will help you create a strong, positive foundation that will help you achieve your health and weight-loss goals on Beyond Diet.

Clear Your Mind

To truly be successful with Beyond Diet, you must clear your mind of all media information and hype. This means not believing everything you hear from so-called health and nutrition experts on TV and radio and in magazines and books. Forget all the other diets that you've tried, and remember that this plan isn't anything like those diets—it's a program that will help you lose weight while improving your overall health. If old habits keep bringing you to the same place—overweight, unhealthy, and unhappy—then you must change your approach.

Believe in What You Are Doing

For this program to be successful, you must believe in yourself. You can change your habits. You can feel great. And you can change the state of your health and weight. Forget all those times you tried different diets. This is a new day and a new approach. This time, it's about overall health.

When you begin to make any lifestyle change, you will encounter people who will try to sabotage your healthy habits in an effort to make themselves feel better. You know the people I'm talking about—the ones who say, "Oh, one won't kill you" or "Eating like that is no way to live." Well, feeling horrible each day, jeopardizing your health by carrying excess weight, not being able to keep up with your children or grandchildren, and avoiding certain activities because of your weight is no way to live. Truly believe in your new way of life and what you are doing for yourself, and don't let anyone tell you otherwise.

Eliminate Negative Thinking

Similarly, you need to free yourself from any negative thinking. If you've thought before, "What's the use? I'll only gain it back anyway," stop right there. You're through with the dieting game. Those negative thoughts are thoughts that the old you would have had, not the new, healthier you. From this point on, replace each negative thought with a positive one. The second you find yourself thinking, "I know I'm going to fail," tell yourself, "I know I can successfully change my eating habits and my life." If you repeat this statement at least five times a day, or simply use it to replace any negative thinking, I guarantee that you will begin to feel more positive and confident about your efforts to adopt a new lifestyle.

Commit Yourself to Doing the Work

Think about your biggest accomplishment to date. What did it take for you to achieve that goal? Months of overtime making yourself eligible for a job promotion? Countless hours helping your child learn a new skill? Years of practice to become successful at a sport or hobby? Accomplishment requires a great deal of work, commitment, and dedication. Achieving your health and lifestyle goals will require work. But as you know from experience, the results are worth it.

Set Goals and Positive Affirmations

Before you start the food and lifestyle changes outlined in this manual, choose three affirmations, which essentially are statements that will help you feel your best. Repeat these statements a minimum of five times per day—not out loud, so that the next person in the Shop Rite line thinks you've lost it, but to yourself—maybe in the morning as you brush your hair, in the car as you drive to work, in the afternoon as you run errands, and at night before you go to bed. The more often, the better. These statements will make you feel so good, you'll be motivated to stick with your new eating habits.

Imagine how great you'd feel if you said affirmations like these to yourself throughout the day:

- *I am a confident, disciplined person and can achieve anything I want.*

- *Eating fresh, wholesome food makes me look and feel great.*

- *I love my life, and every day of it is a blessing.*

The best way to choose your own affirmations is to choose three or more goals, and then turn them into positive statements. For example, if one of your goals is to find the time to exercise more often, then one of your positive affirmations might be, "I have enough time in my day to take care of my health." Choose three important personal goals, and create three positive affirmations for yourself. After you have chosen your affirmations, write them on an index card, and carry the card with you everywhere you go.

My index card of affirmations is in my wallet. I choose not to show it to anybody, but if I have any negative thoughts during the day, I quickly pull it out and repeat my affirmations as many times as it takes to get me out of that negative mind-set. I also repeat my affirmations first thing in the morning and last thing at night. This way, I start and end my day feeling positive and inspired!

A few other ideas:

- Make extra copies of your affirmations, and leave them in places where they will remind you to repeat them during the day (e.g., in the book you're currently reading, in a desk drawer, in the kitchen).

- Tape a copy of your affirmations to the bathroom mirror, so you can give yourself a pep talk while you brush your teeth.

- Add your affirmations to your Success Journal.

Believe me when I tell you that without positive affirmations, my own journey to health would not have been possible. This single step has helped me and thousands of Beyond Diet members achieve their weight loss and lifestyle goals.

2: Three Steps to Weight Loss

Believe it or not, weight loss success is only three steps away! It might not be a quick-and-easy fix, but I promise you that it is possible and that you can do it with the guidance presented in this manual.

To be successful with Beyond Diet, you will have to do some work. This work entails many small tasks that essentially can be grouped in three main steps: Determine your metabolism type, create your personal meal plan, and learn which healthy foods you should choose.

After you have completed these three steps, you will have all the tools you need to achieve the long-term results you desire: weight loss and optimum health for life.

Step 1: Determine Your Metabolism Type

Just as you are unique in all other respects, your body's biochemistry requires certain types and proportions of healthy proteins, carbohydrates, and fats to perform optimally. This unique makeup is called your metabolism type. Learning your metabolism type will help you to lose weight in a safe and healthy manner, once and for all, and achieve optimum wellness. It will also help you achieve long-term results without the starvation and cravings that usually accompany most other diet plans. What's more, it's easy to do with the questionnaire that you will complete with your Metabolism Type Test. Take the Metabolism Type Test online at http://www.beyonddiet.com/Members/Tools/MetabolismType.

Although volumes have been written to explain this step, you only need to know the basics to get started:

- In general, everyone is a Carb Type, a Protein Type, or a Mixed Type. Each type requires ideal amounts and varieties of healthy proteins, carbohydrates, and fats (which will be explained in the Chapter on Meal Planning).

- Requirements for the appropriate ratios and types of healthy proteins, carbohydrates, and fats exist along a fixed spectrum. The requirements for people whose biochemistries require high amounts of protein for optimal health (Protein Types) are located at one end, and those for people whose biochemistries demand high amounts of healthy carbohydrates (Carb Types) are at the other end. Mixed Types are a combination of these two types, so their requirements fall somewhere in the middle.

- Medical doctors and nutrition pioneers have used metabolism typing for decades. It has helped people not only experience dramatic weight loss but also overcome severe chronic disease, obesity, and other serious disorders.

Learning your metabolism type will help you answer many common dietary mysteries that you have always wondered about:

- Why can some people be successful—at least in losing weight over the short term—on popular low-carbohydrate, low-fat, or other diets while many others fail miserably on the same diets? Because success with any diet depends on the dieter's metabolism type; in other words, the same-diet-for-everyone approach simply is not effective.

- How can one kind of food be so good for one person—giving energy and apparent health—but affect someone else in a completely different way, making them tired and cranky? Because certain foods are ideal for each metabolism type. Just because a food is considered healthy in general does not mean that it's healthy for everyone.

Learning your metabolism type is essential to creating the meal plans that will work best for you. The ideal foods (and the ratios in which you should eat them) for your metabolism type will create the foundation for your personal meal plan. Internationally renowned natural health expert and advocate Joseph Mercola, D.O. (2005), uses metabolism typing with all of his patients for weight loss and to alleviate disease symptoms.

Weight Loss vs. Fat Loss

Losing weight and losing fat are not the same thing. To look and feel your best, you should lose weight specifically from body fat, not from muscle.

Studies often find that two groups of people consuming the same amount of calories but in different ratios of proteins, carbohydrates, and fats will lose different amounts of body fat and lean body mass (e.g., muscle and bone). For instance, someone who is a Protein Type but eats a 1,500-calorie diet composed of mostly carbohydrates each day most likely will not lose weight—or worse, may gain weight. On a 1,500-calorie diet of mostly protein, some carbohydrates, and healthy fats, this same person will reach his or her weight loss goal and feel great! (Discover the optimum food ratios for you in the Chapter on Daily Meal Planning.)

To lose weight from fat, you must focus on not only how many calories you consume but also the source of those calories (i.e., proteins, carbohydrates, or fats). Eating the foods that are ideal for your metabolism type greatly affects the source of your weight loss. When your hormones are in balance (because you're eating what your body requires), your body will achieve its ideal metabolic rate and will not need to hold onto excess fat stores—and as a result, weight loss will come from stored fat.

To conceptualize this situation, imagine yourself outside in freezing winter weather, dressed in a winter parka. If you entered a warm shelter, you would remove your coat because it would no longer be needed. The parka is like stored body fat: necessary under certain conditions but not others.

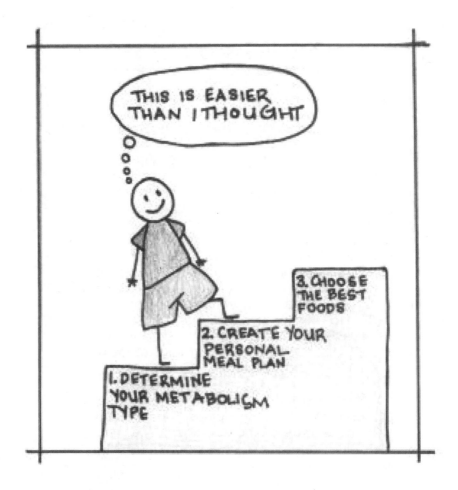

Step 2: Create Your Personal Meal Plan

Knowing your metabolism type, you will be able to tap into the wealth of resources needed to create a personal meal plan that will allow you to achieve long-term weight loss and optimum health. In the Chapter on Calories, you will estimate healthy daily calorie requirements for achieving and maintaining your ideal weight. Using your Success Journal, you will record your daily food intake and track how you feel afterward. Finally, the Chapter on Daily Meal Planning will guide you in choosing the ideal foods for your metabolism type, in the ideal proportions and serving sizes, and creating your own meal plan.

All of the resources you need in order to choose, combine, and portion your food properly are included in this manual and your bonus materials. The numerous charts show you the ideal ratios of proteins, carbohydrates, and fats for your metabolism type; which foods are the best choices for your metabolism type; and how to build a meal plan that takes all this personal information into account.

Step 3: Choose the Best Foods

The third, and maybe most important, step toward weight loss and overall health is to identify which foods to eat. To save yourself a lot of time, just follow this guideline: If it's natural—that is, it grows, or otherwise occurs, in nature—eat it; if it's artificial, don't. In other words, if a food contains ingredients that you can't pronounce or define, steer clear.

Natural foods span all the food groups and include fresh, unprocessed fruits and vegetables; unroasted tree nuts and ground nuts; whole seeds and grains; and unadulterated fats, dairy, and meat products. Foods in the artificial category include packaged foods, frozen meals, cookies and cakes, artificial sweeteners (e.g., saccharin [Sweet'N Low], aspartame [NutraSweet], and sucralose [Splenda]), hydrogenated oils (e.g., margarine and Crisco), high-fructose corn syrup, and any prepared products that contain any of these ingredients.

To understand why this distinction is important, you must understand the function of the liver. The liver is the body's largest internal organ, and it's responsible for an astonishing variety of life-sustaining and health-promoting tasks, including those that make healthy weight loss and weight management possible. Integral to countless metabolic processes, the liver supports the digestive system, controls blood sugar, and regulates fat storage. One of the liver's most important functions—and the one most crucial to weight loss—is the chemical breakdown of everything that enters your body.

It is the liver's job to distinguish between the nutrients to be absorbed and the dangerous or unnecessary substances to be filtered out of the bloodstream. But when overwhelmed with toxins (like artificial sweeteners and other chemicals that are added to packaged foods), the liver gets "clogged" and cannot effectively process nutrients and fats. If your liver cannot process the nutrients and fats that your body needs, you will gain weight and won't be able to lose it.

The liver also produces bile, a substance crucial to the detoxification of the body. Bile helps break down fats and assimilate fat-soluble vitamins. But when bile becomes overly congested with the toxins it's trying to filter out, it simply can't function properly. It becomes thick, viscous, and highly inefficient.

What qualifies as a toxin? Anything that your body does not recognize as a food source. Artificial sweeteners, for example, have zero calories because the body does not recognize them as food sources. But they still have to pass through the liver, as do other synthetic ingredients that you can't even pronounce.

Food-processing chemicals and other toxins also irritate the gastrointestinal system, which may manifest as bloating, constipation, or gas in many people. Chronic constipation may also lead to difficulty losing weight, not to mention a long list of other harmful health problems.

Toxins are stored in fat cells—that is, they are embedded in body fat. The more fat in your body, the more toxins you can store. Stored toxins cause your cells and organs to become sluggish and inefficient. Toxins also attack and destroy cells and gene structures. They create an acidic environment in the body that is vulnerable to fungi, bacteria, parasites, worms, viruses, and many other pathogens. Organs and body systems under a toxic load lose their ability to metabolize and process fat effectively.

The body stores toxins in fat tissue. In fact, toxin storage is one of the main functions of fat stores; this protective mechanism keeps toxins away from vital organs. When you ingest fewer toxins, your body will not need as much fat to store them and will quickly begin to let go of excess fat. This process leads to not only the right kind of weight loss (from fat) but also a healthy, disease-free body.

The body also stores toxins wherever it is weak. This makes the weak area even weaker and eventually can manifest in a cyst or disease. An area left diseased for too long becomes difficult to repair. To achieve an ideal weight and healthy body, it is vital to eat only clean, unprocessed food from this point forward.

3: Metabolism Types

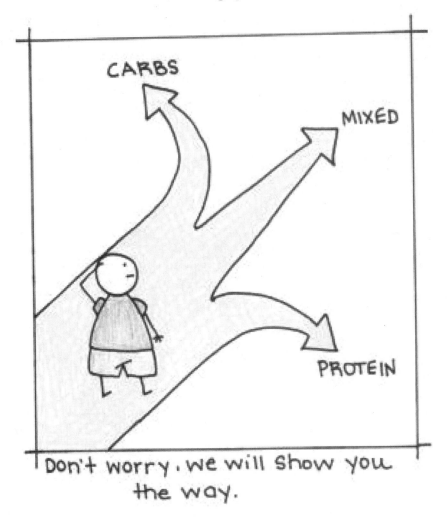

Please complete the Metabolism Type Test on Beyond Diet to determine your metabolism type —Protein Type, Carb Type, or Mixed Type. Next, read through the description of (and special considerations for) your metabolism type in this chapter. You must understand why certain foods are ideal in order to make the best choices for your personal meal plan.

As you learn about your metabolism type in this chapter, remember that each person is unique, so some fine-tuning may be necessary as you change your eating habits. Pay close attention to your body's cues. Most people have fallen out of touch with their bodies and don't know what true health feels like. Pay close attention to the one and only source that knows what's best for you—your body!

Protein Types

Protein Types typically crave rich, fatty foods such as pizza, sausages, and salty roasted nuts. They love food, may not feel satiated after a snack, and often feel hungry, even after eating a large meal. When they have eaten too many carbohydrates, Protein Types tend to crave sugar. And once they start eating sugary foods, they want more and more and may find it difficult to stop. Sugar often causes Protein Types to feel jittery and will quickly make their energy levels drop.

Protein Types may have tried to lose weight by using extreme calorie-cutting methods, only to be unsuccessful—and feel miserable in the process. Protein Types cannot successfully lose weight by drastically decreasing calorie intake.

When Protein Types eat the wrong kind of food, they may notice energy problems—extreme fatigue or a wired "on edge" feeling. Eating often makes them feel better when they feel anxious, nervous, or shaky, but then they feel worse soon afterward. These cycles of energy ups and downs are definite signs of a mismatch between metabolism type and food consumption.

What Does a Protein Type Need?

Protein Types need a diet high in proteins and fats and low in carbohydrates. But think balance—not the Atkins Diet! Protein Types can eat various carbohydrates in the form of some grains, fruits, and vegetables, as long as they are adequately balanced with proteins and fats.

Because Protein Types metabolize food more quickly than other metabolism types (which is why they feel hungry all the time), heavier protein choices such as whole eggs, dark-meat poultry, beef, and dairy are essential for ideal meal planning. These foods have long been considered "unhealthy" because of their high fat content, but as you will learn in the Chapter on Fats, saturated fat is not the cause of disease; refined carbohydrates, processed foods, and hydrogenated oils are. Protein Types who do not eat heavy proteins with a high fat content will be hungry all day and struggle with their weight. Even worse, they will almost always feel fatigued and anxious.

"Must Do's" for Protein Types

- **Eat protein at every meal and with every snack.** Eating only carbohydrates at a meal causes blood sugar to spike and then drop quickly, which will leave a Protein Type feeling hungry, fatigued, and anxious as well as cause cravings for more carbohydrates shortly afterward. Eating protein— especially animal protein—at every meal and for snacks will help to control blood sugar levels and leave Protein Types feeling satiated and steady throughout the day. *Remember to listen to your body—pay attention to which meals and snacks leave you hungry or craving more.*

- **Eat small meals frequently or healthy snacks between meals.** Protein Types need to eat often; otherwise, they'll suffer from extremely low blood sugar levels. Going too long between meals (or snacks) also will create ravenous hunger, which in turn will cause overeating at the next meal—only to lead to lethargy and an uncomfortable feeling afterward.

- **Avoid refined carbohydrates.** Foods such as bread, crackers, and pastas—especially those made from wheat— can be extremely disruptive for Protein Types. Wheat breaks down into sugar faster than any other grain and causes the rapid release of large quantities of insulin. That is why sprouted whole grain bread products are the only allowable sources of bread. These products are described in the

Chapter on Grains.

- **Avoid most fruits and fruit juices.** Fruits are a wonderful, healthy food, but Protein Types need to be extra careful with their fruit selections. Some fruits are quickly converted to sugar in the bloodstream and cause extreme blood sugar fluctuations. The best fruit choices for Protein Types are apples and avocados (high in fiber and low in sugar). Some people may be able to eat more of these fruits than others.

Carb Types

Carb Types tend to have weak appetites. They tend to be happy with a minimal amount of food each day and can get by on small amounts of food. Carb Types don't give food much thought until they feel hungry.

Carb Types tend to eat less often because they "have no time to eat." These goal-oriented workaholics will skip meals to do what they need to do each day. They may go for extended periods without eating, sending the metabolism into starvation mode. Decreasing the metabolic rate in this fashion can lead to weight management problems and obesity. Carb Types also are more dependent on caffeinated beverages to get them through the day than other metabolism types are. This dependency often weakens their appetites even more, compounding their nutritional problems.

Carb Types have a high tolerance for baked goods and starchy vegetables. This can be a bad thing, because they tend to overeat these carbohydrates, which can lead to unhealthy conditions such as hypoglycemia, insulin resistance, and diabetes.

What Does a Carb Type Need?

A Carb Type needs a diet composed of more carbohydrates than proteins or fats. But that doesn't mean that Carb Types don't need protein throughout the day. Lighter, low-fat proteins such as white-meat poultry and whitefish (e.g., tilapia, sea bass) are good choices. Carb Types can choose from a wide variety of carbohydrates and can eat them in larger quantities than any other type.

Although Carb Types convert carbohydrates into energy slowly (unlike Protein Types), it does not mean that they can go on carbohydrate binges. An elevated insulin response is still a concern, especially if weight loss is the goal. Insulin is a fat-storing hormone, so large quantities in the bloodstream will make losing weight quite difficult. Remember, excess of any particular food can lead to weight gain and disease, so always maintain the food portions and ratios recommended for your type (according to the **Ideal Food Ratios For Each Metabolism Type Chart**).

Carb Types lose weight and feel well on a high-carbohydrate, low-fat diet—the opposite of what a Protein Type needs.

"Must Do's" for Carb Types

- **Choose low-fat proteins.** Incorporate a low-fat protein such as white-meat poultry or whitefish into each meal. Avoid (or eat only occasionally) high-fat proteins, which may cause lethargy, depression, or fatigue.

- **Choose dairy products carefully.** Carb Types tend to metabolize dairy poorly. The best way to learn whether dairy is a wise choice is to carefully monitor the body's reaction after consuming it with a meal. If you feel lethargic or fatigued shortly after, limit your dairy consumption.

- **Choose carbohydrates carefully.** Choose plenty of low-starch vegetables, like broccoli and salad greens, and limit consumption of high-starch foods such as bread, pasta, and grains. Eating too many grains may result in feeling sluggish, sleepy, or hungry soon after a meal containing a low-fat protein, a vegetable, and a grain. Try increasing the protein amount and decreasing the grain amount the next time you have this same meal.

- **Monitor your response to legumes.** Carb Types typically cannot easily digest the type of protein that most legumes contain. Therefore, eat legumes infrequently. As with all other foods, monitor the body's response carefully, and pay attention to its ability to combine them with certain foods. Some people can eat chicken, beans, and vegetables and feel great, but feel tired and sluggish if they eat beans, rice, and vegetables.

- **Limit the nuts and seeds.** Carb Types feel best on a low-fat diet, and nuts and seeds add too much fat to a meal. Nuts and nut butters are great protein choices for snacks, but lean animal meats are better protein choices for meals.

Mixed Types

A Mixed Type requires an equal balance of proteins, carbohydrates, and healthy fats, and including variety in the everyday meal plan is essential. Of the three metabolism types, this one is actually easiest to manage, because the food choices are greater. Some meals may resemble those for Protein Types, and some may resemble those for Carb Types; some may have features of both.

The appetite of a Mixed Type tends to vary greatly throughout the day—hungry at meals but not in between, ravenous at times and no appetite at others. Of course, these responses depend on what foods have been eaten that day. Mixed Types generally don't suffer from cravings. However, like the other types, Mixed Types who eat too much sugar or too many carbohydrates may develop strong sugar cravings.

Mixed Types must incorporate high-fat and low-fat proteins, as well as high-starch and low-starch carbohydrates, into their meal plans. As a Mixed Type, it is important to be familiar with the requirements of both types to find the perfect balance.

A Mixed Type may be more of a Protein Mixed Type or a Carb Mixed

Type—in other words, have more qualities of one type than the other. The only way to truly figure this out is by trial and error: by paying close attention to the body's responses to each meal, Mixed Types can determine which foods make them feel good and energized and which foods leave them feeling hungry, fatigued, cranky, or craving more. Finding the right balance of proteins, carbohydrates, and fats is the key to losing weight, feeling great, and achieving optimal health.

4: Calories

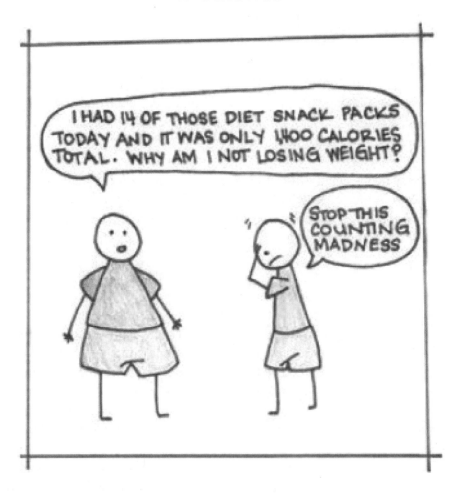

When most people think about weight loss and daily food consumption, the first word that comes to mind is *calorie.* In my experience, the mere mention of the word makes most people go pale, but at the same time, many people simply don't know what it means. For this reason, I would eliminate *calorie* from the English language if I could. The word is not bad in and of itself, but it is widely misunderstood!

In this chapter, I will present the facts about calories so you can be in-the-know. Then, I will clarify some common misconceptions about what calories are and what calories do so you can make healthy decisions about how and what to eat. Finally, you will use an easy equation to estimate your daily calorie requirements to lose weight or maintain it. Then you can forget about counting calories forever. (Really!)

Learn the Facts

According to *Merriam-Webster's Collegiate Dictionary* (11th edition), a *calorie* is "a unit equivalent to the large calorie expressing heat-producing or energy-producing value in food when oxidized in the body." In plain English, a *calorie* is a unit of energy that is released from the food you eat and used to power the body.

The body needs energy from food—calories—to perform many functions, the most obvious of which are exercise and other kinds of physical activity. However, the body also requires energy to function at the most basic level: to breathe, digest food, and maintain organs and organ systems.

Believe it or not, it is possible to eat too few calories! The most serious problem with low-calorie diets is that although they may bring about weight loss, they also can cause serious health problems. One common side effect of low-calorie diets is muscle breakdown, which can occur when the body doesn't receive enough calories from protein. Especially vulnerable is the heart, a muscular organ. If a person does not consume an adequate amount of calories each day, the heart muscle begins to break down, possibly leading to serious conditions such as cardiac atrophy.

Also, following low-calorie diets off and on over time can have negative consequences for overall health. Low-calorie diets typically do not supply enough energy to keep organs and systems healthy and, in effect, can lead to malnourishment. For clients who have repeatedly followed such diets, I recommend high-calorie meal plans that provide their organs with adequate fuel to repair themselves and regain health.

End the Calorie Debate

The American public has been told, time and time again, that consuming more calories than the body burns leads to weight gain. However, this statement is only partially true. In the following sections, I will clear up some common misconceptions about calories.

"A calorie is a calorie."

The old school of nutritional thinking teaches that all calories are created equal. Weight loss and weight gain are strictly a matter of "calories in, calories out": Regardless of the calorie source, you'll lose weight if you burn more calories than you eat and gain weight if you eat more calories than you burn.

This explanation seems logical enough, right? Unfortunately, it fails to account for modern research findings that the calories from proteins, carbohydrates, and fats have different effects on body metabolism—in other words, some calories really are healthier than others. To grasp this concept, a basic understanding of metabolism is helpful.

Two important metabolic reactions involve insulin and glucagon, hormones that are released during the digestion of food consumed. In general, *insulin* causes fat storage, and *glucagon* causes fat to be used for energy (rather than stored). The body needs both of these hormones so it can function properly, but when the insulin–glucagon balance is ideal, the body will actually build muscle while burning fat. Getting the proportions correct is key to achieving and maintaining a healthy weight, and eating the right foods for your unique metabolism type—regardless of the calorie content of those foods—is the best way to do that.

Certain foods affect insulin release much more than other foods. These foods are refined carbohydrates, which include white breads, sugars, most baked goods, and most processed snack foods. Consuming such foods causes insulin levels to increase quickly (giving a short, high energy boost) and then decrease quickly (leading to low energy levels and listlessness). When your body releases too much insulin, you may feel hungry soon after eating. Conversely, protein causes the release of glucagon, which can decrease hunger and control appetite.

By the way, it also is incorrect to say that all fats—or carbohydrates, or proteins—are created equal. Different fats (e.g., fish oil vs. hydrogenated oil) have vastly different effects on metabolism and health in general, as do different carbohydrates (e.g., low glycemic index vs. high glycemic index) and different proteins (animal vs. plant). The differences are highlighted throughout this manual.

As you see, making educated choices about where your calories come from is important when you are attempting to control appetite, lose weight, or maintain a healthy weight in the long term.

"Calories don't matter."

This school of thought says that if you eat proteins, carbohydrates, and fats in certain ratios, then the number of calories is unimportant. For example, for proponents of metabolism typing, the only thing that matters is eating the ideal foods in the right proportions for your metabolism type. This approach can be effective if you eat those foods in the ideal amounts for your body; however, consuming larger amounts will cause you to maintain or gain weight rather than lose it.

If a meal plan for weight loss isn't created with calorie counts, then on what is it based? Ideally, each of us would know when to eat and when to stop eating simply by "listening" to the body's hunger and satiation cues. Unfortunately, though, most people who struggle with their weight have lost the ability to recognize when they are hungry or full and often eat when they feel stressed, bored, or pressured socially.

There is a way to account for this inability to listen to the body's cues, though. Estimate how many calories you need to consume daily (Determine Daily Calorie Requirements, later in this chapter - you can also do this on Beyond Diet) and then use the result as a tool to determine ideal serving sizes (Step 2: Determine Your Allowable Food Servings, in the **Chapter on Daily Meal Planning**, as well as on Beyond Diet). Then, by paying attention to your body's cues over time, you can create and adjust future meal plans accordingly.

"I can't eat that much and still lose weight."

Many people are surprised by the generous portion sizes and the amounts of food that this program recommends for healthy weight loss. But the truth is, with the right foods, you can eat sizable quantities of food and lose weight at the same time! Most dieters decrease their food intake so much when they want to lose weight that they do lose some pounds [kilos], then quickly plateau. At that point, they have no recourse but to eat even less food, which triggers starvation mode and makes losing weight and feeling good difficult, if not impossible.

Please don't be afraid to eat. If you eat the right foods, in the right amounts and proportions for your metabolism type, then you will lose weight and feel great. You must change your mind-set from "calorie counting" to "choosing the appropriate proportions and serving sizes" for your body. And whatever you do, don't be lured into the trap of counting calories, because that approach is not sustainable—or healthy—in the long term.

Determine Daily Calorie Requirements

Even though the word *calorie* is loaded with bad (and wrong) connotations, this program suggests estimating your daily calorie requirements as a means to an end. This number is used to determine the correct number of servings of each food type for each meal (Step 2: Determine Your Allowable Food Servings). That's it—no counting calories at each meal, or ever! (In fact, for my clients, I always did the calorie calculation myself and chose the appropriate meal plan without ever mentioning the word *calorie*.) Instead, you will use your **Success Journal** to record the individual servings of proteins, carbohydrates, and fats that you consume at each meal and your total servings for each day. A great way to keep track of all of these is in your online Success Journal on Beyond Diet.

How many calories are enough—that is, enough to provide energy for your body to perform all its necessary functions and activities and bring about optimum health? Daily calorie requirements vary from person to person and depend on weight, foods consumed, sleep, stress and activity levels, age, and a long list of other factors that affect metabolism. Because of these many variables, no machine, calculator, or equation can determine the exact number of calories that a person needs daily. However, my experience indicates that the following calorie equation provides a good starting point, even if it is not the most scientific method.

Read the following instructions straight through once, then perform the easy calculation for yourself, recording your results here. You will need to refer to this information while you work through the **Chapter on Daily Meal Planning.** You can also use the online Caloric Calculator (located at http://www.beyonddiet.com/Members/Tools/CaloricCalculator)— simply input your weight and choose your activity level, and your daily requirement will be calculated for you.

- Multiply your current weight (in pounds) by 13, 14, or 15 [weight (in kilograms) by 28.6, 30.7, or 33]—use 13 [28.6] if you have a particularly slow metabolism and do not exercise much, 14 [30.7] if you perform moderate exercise three or more times per week, and 15 [33] if you exercise vigorously more than three times per week. The result is your *daily calorie requirement for weight maintenance:*

  _____ pounds [kilos] × ___ = _____ calories per day

- For healthy weight loss, you must reduce your maintenance calorie intake by 20% (in other words, consume 80% of the maintenance amount). Simply multiply your daily calorie requirement for weight maintenance by 0.80. (**Note:** Do not reduce your calories by more than 20% in an effort to lose more weight; doing so may put your body in a starvation state, which would slow your metabolism and make weight loss even more difficult). The result is your *daily calorie requirement to achieve healthy weight loss*:

  _____ calories × 0.80 = _____ calories per day

For example, consider a 180-pound [80-kg] female who does moderate weight training and walking three times per week.

Maintenance plan:

180 pounds × 14 = 2,520 calories per day
(80 kilograms × 30.7 = 2,456 calories per day)

Weight-loss plan:

2,520 calories × 0.80 = 2,016 calories per day
(2,456 calories × 0.80 = 1,965 calories per day)

Her customized weight-loss meal plan should provide about 2,000 calories per day.

Remember that these daily calorie requirements are only guidelines. Some people need fewer calories to lose weight, and others need more. The goal is to consume as many calories as possible while still losing fat, because the more fuel you give the body, the harder your metabolism will work, and you want to keep that metabolism cranking to see long-term weight loss. The truth is, the healthier your body is, the more food you can eat and still achieve or maintain your ideal weight. Calculate your daily calorie requirements online at BeyondDiet.com.

Frequently Asked Questions

What if my calorie requirements are above 2400 calories?

If your calorie requirement totals an amount above 2400 calories, begin on the 2400 calorie meal plan as your baseline serving amounts. Let your body dictate whether you need to add more or less to your plan. If you are experiencing hunger after the first 3 days, add 1-2 servings of protein, 1-2 servings of fat, and/or 1-2 servings of carbohydrate to your daily meal plan.

I want to gain weight. How do my calculations change?

If healthy weight gain is your goal, you will want to adjust your calorie calculations. Instead of subtracting 20% from your baseline calories, you will add 20%. For example, a very active male who wishes to gain weight, primarily in the form of muscle, would multiply his current weight by 15, multiply this number by 20%, and then add that total to the initial calorie calculation.

5: Daily Meal Planning

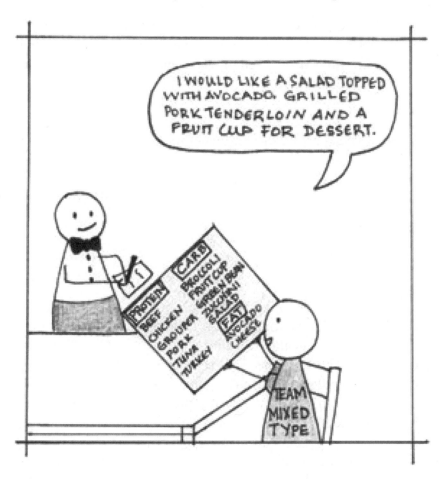

Now you have almost all the information and tools you need to begin to create your personal meal plan. In this chapter, you will learn the proper food ratios for your metabolism type, determine the ideal food servings for your daily calorie requirements, refine the food choices for your metabolism type, and then use all of this information to create your own personal meal plan—and be well on your way to weight loss success.

At this point, you should have already discovered whether you are a Protein Type, a Carb Type, or a Mixed Type according to the instructions in the **Chapter on Metabolism Types** or using the Metabolism Type Test on BeyondDiet.com; estimated your daily calorie requirements using the equation in the **Chapter on Calories** or the Caloric Calculator on BeyondDiet.com; and printed your **Success Journal** (or located it on BeyondDiet.com). We'll use the following charts in the **Guides and Charts Chapter** (towards the end of this manual) to create your meal plans in your **Success Journal**:

- Allowable Servings Chart
- Ideal Food Ratios For Each Metabolism Type Chart
- Food Choices Chart

Step 1: Identify Ideal Protein– Carbohydrate–Fat Ratios

On the Ideal Food Ratios for Each Metabolism Type chart, you see that different ratios of calories from proteins, carbohydrates (listed as Carbs on the chart), and fats are ideal for each metabolism type. Carb Types should eat approximately 20% proteins, 70% carbohydrates, and 10% fats; Mixed Types should eat approximately 40% proteins, 50% carbohydrates, and 10% fats; and Protein Types should eat approximately 45% proteins, 35% carbohydrates, and 20% fats.

For example, if you're a Mixed Type, each meal or snack (including your drink) should contain about half protein and half carbohydrates. (**Note:** The 10% fat would come from your protein source or from some added healthy oil.) Use the **Allowable Servings Guide** to create your own meal plans. You'll soon learn to tune in to your body's responses and learn when you have eaten the right amounts for you.

Step 2: Determine Your Allowable Food Servings

To determine your ideal food servings, refer to the **Allowable Servings Guide**. Locate the heading that lists your daily calorie requirements (as determined by the calorie equation given under Determine Daily Calorie Requirements, in the **Chapter on Calories**), then the column in that section that applies to your metabolism type. For example, a person who requires 2,000 calories a day and is a Protein Type should search first for the "2,000 calories/day" heading (bottom left section of the chart) and then for the Protein information (unshaded column under the "2,000 calories/day" heading). Starting from the top of this column, you can see that this person should have three protein servings and one carbohydrate serving for Breakfast, three protein servings and one carbohydrate serving for a Snack, and so on down the column.

Transfer your allowable servings information to a new page in your **Success Journal**.

After completing the Caloric Calculator and Metabolism Type Test on BeyondDiet.com, you can also access your Allowable Servings: http://www.beyonddiet.com/Members/Tools/FoodServings. These servings will automatically be updated in your online Success Journal.

Step 3: Identify Your Ideal Foods

Eating the right kinds of food is just as important as eating the right quantities of food. Take a look at the **Food Choices** charts for your metabolism type (e.g., a Protein Type would use the Protein chart, and Carb Type would use the Carbohydrate chart; a Mixed Type would use the Mixed chart). These can be found in the Charts section of this manual, as well as online at http://www.beyonddiet.com/Members/Food. The ideal foods for each type are shaded in the appropriate charts. Foods that are not highlighted in the charts should be avoided or eaten only occasionally. For example, an orange—generally thought of as a healthy food—will help balance a Carb Type but may push a Protein Type out of balance.

Because each person is unique, these charts must be considered as a starting point to find which foods are best for you. For example, I always test as a Protein Type but feel pretty good eating cucumbers and carrots—two foods that most Protein Types typically should avoid. When I feel lethargic soon after eating or hungry an hour later, I know I've eaten a food that isn't good for me (or that my meal didn't have the correct protein-to-carbohydrate ratio).

Again, these charts are only starting points to determine which foods might be best for you. Pay attention to how you feel after eating; track symptoms that might be related to the foods you eat in your **Success Journal**.

Step 4: Plan Your Meals

Finally, put all the pieces together to create a truly personal meal plan—one that meets the needs of your metabolism type and includes foods that you enjoy. Let's start with an example.

According to the **Allowable Servings Guide**, a Protein Type requires three protein servings at Breakfast. Possible options from the Protein Type chart could be

- 2 eggs and 1 slice of bacon

- 3 ounces [84 g] of meat or poultry (possibly leftovers from the night before)

- or something else from the chart

A Protein Type also requires one carbohydrate serving at Breakfast. Possible options from the Carbohydrate chart could be

- 1 medium apple

- 1 cup [180 g] of spinach (e.g., in an omelet)

- 1 cup [150 g] of cooked oatmeal

- or something else from the chart

For a Snack, a Protein Type requires three protein servings and one carbohydrate serving, which could be

- 1½ ounces [42 g] of raw almonds and 1 medium apple

- 3 oz [84 g] leftover turkey and ½ cup [75 g] each of celery and carrots

- or something else from the chart

Now plan a Breakfast using your unique information, and list these choices on a Meal Planning worksheet in your **Success Journal** under Breakfast. Refer to the example Meal Plans provided below. (Although the serving sizes may not be exact for your needs, the sample meals demonstrate how to combine servings of proteins, carbohydrates, and fats together in a meal.) You can also plan your meals in your online Success Journal: http://www.beyonddiet.com/Members/Journal

Do the same thing for your morning and afternoon Snacks. Keep in mind that snacks don't have to be the kinds of unhealthy, empty-calorie foods that people normally associate with snacking (chips, candy, and cookies). Healthy, nutritious snack alternatives like raw nuts and a fruit also have the advantage of being easily transportable. To choose your best snack options, think about your typical day and where you will be during mid-morning and mid-afternoon snack times. If you will be on the move, then your snack should be shelf-stable, easily transportable, and easy to eat with your hands. If you will have access to a refrigerator or a cooler, then your snack can be a mini meal that consists of leftovers from the day before.

The process of creating meals for Lunch and Dinner is the same as for Breakfast and Snacks, but you will add Fat servings, as indicated on the **Allowable Servings Guide**. Don't give in to society's urging to avoid all fats, thinking that doing so will help you lose weight faster. In fact, you must consume a substantial amount of healthy fat each day to lose weight, keep energy levels high, and feel satiated. (the **Chapter on Fats** addresses this topic in detail.) You can also look through the **Recipe Guide** and the Recipes section of Beyond Diet (http://www.beyonddiet.com/Members/Recipes) to help you cook up some healthy and delicious meals.

5: Daily Meal Planning

Plan another day or two of meals while you're at it, using another page in your **Success Journal** or online at http://www.beyonddiet.com/Members/ Tools/FoodServings.

Here are examples of what a daily meal plan may look like for each Metabolism Type:

Sample Meal Plan- Protein Type				
Food		**Servings**		
Qty	**Item**	**P**	**C**	**F**
	BREAKFAST			
3 oz	Lamb, Chicken, or Turkey sausage	3		
1 cup	Mushrooms and spinach		1	
	Coconut oil			
	SNACK			
1 cup	Sliced celery and carrots		1	
3 Tbsp	Walnut butter	3		
	LUNCH			
5 oz	Beef burger	5		
1 cup	Spinach salad with celery, cauliflower and cucumbers		1	
	Apple cider vinegar and 2 tsp olive oil			2
	SNACK			
1 small	Green apple		1	
3	Hardboiled eggs	3		
	DINNER			
5 oz	Beef steak	5		
1 cup	Steamed carrots and cauliflower		1	
2 tsp	Butter			2

Sample Meal Plan- Carb Type				
Food		**Servings**		
Qty	**Item**	**P**	**C**	**F**
	BREAKFAST			
2	Turkey or chicken breakfast sausage	2		
1 cup	Green beans or spaghetti squash		1	
1 cup	Strawberries		2	
	SNACK			
1/2 oz	Pumpkin seeds	1		
1	Banana		1	
	LUNCH			
3 oz	Mahi mahi (broiled)	3		
	Romaine, cucumber and tomato salad		1	
	Apple cider vinegar and 1 tsp olive oil			1
20	Grapes		1	
	SNACK			
1 Tbsp	Almond butter	1		
1	Apple		1	
1/4 cup	Raisins		1	
	DINNER			
3 oz	Cornish hen (baked)	3		
1 cup	Cauliflower (steamed)		1	
1 cup	Broccoli (steamed)		1	
2 tsp	Butter			2
1 cup	Raw red peppers		1	

Sample Meal Plan- Mixed Type				
Food		**Servings**		
Qty	Item	P	C	F
	BREAKFAST			
2	Eggs (omelet)	2		
1 cup	Raw spinach, peppers, onions (omelet)		1	
1 slice	SWG bread		1	
1	Medium pear		1	
	SNACK			
1 oz	Almonds or walnuts	2		
1	Medium apple		1	
1 cup	Cucumber slices		1	
	LUNCH			
4 oz	Turkey, ground white and dark meat (burger)	4		
1 cup	Carrot sticks		1	
1 cup	Small green salad		1	
	Apple cider vinegar + 1 tsp olive oil			1
	SNACK			
1 Tbsp	Almond butter	2		
1 slice	SWG bread		1	
8 oz	Celery sticks		1	
	DINNER			
5 oz	Halibut steak	5		
1/2 cup	Green beans (with garlic)		1/2	
4 oz	Sweet potato		1	
1/2 cup	Small green salad or 1/2 cup raw vegetables		1/2	
	Apple cider vinegar + 1 tsp olive oil			1

Step 5: Learn More

Now that you have planned a few days' worth of Breakfasts, Snacks, Lunches, and Dinners, you are well on your way to achieving your ideal weight and optimum health! Your toolkit is almost complete.

Remember, the information listed in the **Allowable Servings Guide** (http://www.beyonddiet.com/Members/Tools/FoodServings) and **Food Choices** charts (http://www.beyonddiet.com/Members/Food) are only suggestions and starting points. If you feel hungry at any time, you will need to adjust your meal plan in some way. Depending on your metabolism type, you might add a bit more protein, carbohydrate, or fat to a meal (to adjust the protein–carbohydrate–fat ratio slightly) or add another Snack to your day (making sure to keep that meal balanced and appropriate for your type) until you feel satiated and energized. And if something you eat makes you feel lethargic, avoid it.

Likewise, if you feel that the food on your meal plans is too much food for you to eat in one day, you can also modify accordingly. Remember that I don't want you to be hungry, but I also don't want you to spend the day feeling overly full. The portion sizes in the meal plans are designed to give you a sufficient amount of food each day to feel satiated while still burning off unwanted fat. If your lifestyle or body requires less food, modify your meal plans to suit your needs.

Continue reading the rest of the manual so you can learn how to choose the best food available, prepare it in a healthy way, and enjoy your journey toward healthy weight loss. You may want to keep your **Success Journal** handy as you read so that you can make notes to help guide future meal planning.

PART 2

Congratulations on creating your personal meal plan! Take a good look at it. In front of you is the path to your personal weight-loss and health goals.

As important as it is that you eat the foods that are ideal for your metabolism type, it is also critical to choose the best foods possible. This part of the manual is dedicated to teaching you how to choose the foods that will best help you achieve the weight-loss and health goals that your meal plan represents.

6: Organic Food

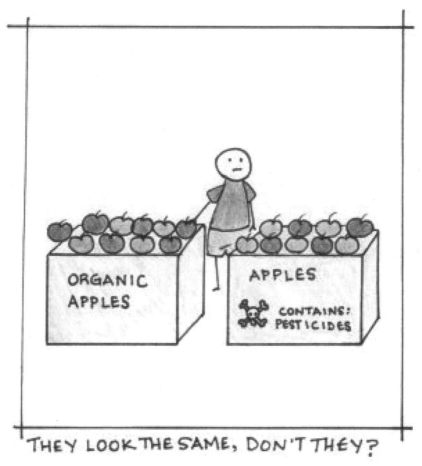

THEY LOOK THE SAME, DON'T THEY?

What exactly is organic food? It is food grown or raised without the use of synthetic (chemically formulated) pesticides, herbicides, fungicides, or fertilizers. Organic farming allows foods to grow in nature as they were intended.

Conventional farmers in the United States alone spray 2 billion pounds [900 million kilos] of pesticides a year on crops to compensate for poor farming practices (Chek 2004, 55). And those pesticides end up in our food supply! In this chapter, I will explain why organic foods are better for your health and should be a part of your healthy lifestyle.

The Truth About Conventional Produce

In *How to Eat, Move and Be Healthy*, Chek (2004) lists the following chemicals found in a conventionally grown apple, a food that most of us would consider healthy!

- Chlorpyrifos: an endocrine disruptor that impairs immune response, causes reproductive abnormalities, and damages a developing nervous system

- Captan: a carcinogen (i.e., a substance believed to be capable of causing cancer) that causes genetic and immune system damage

- Iprodione: a carcinogen

- Vinclozolin: a carcinogen and a genetic, endocrine, and reproductive disruptor that causes dermatitis

Chek also provides the results of an interesting study conducted on 110 urban and suburban children in Washington state. The study found that children who ate primarily organic foods had significantly lower exposure to organophosphorous pesticide (a nervous and immune system disruptor) than children on conventional diets. Of the children tested, only one did not demonstrate measurable pesticide levels in a urine sample; this child ate an all-organic diet. The levels measured in other children who ate mainly organic foods were below the U.S. Environmental Protection Agency's (EPA's) "safe" level, whereas those of children who ate conventional foods were above this level.

Meat, Poultry, and Eggs

The animal that becomes your meal can only be as good and as healthy as the food that it was fed (in the same way that you can only be as healthy as the food you eat: You are what you eat!). In the wild, cattle eat grass, but most commercially raised cattle are fed low-quality grains to make them fat. Because these animals are not designed to eat grains, they quickly become ill, which requires the administration of antibiotics that you ingest when you eat beef.

If this situation is not bad enough, most of the chickens and pigs in commercial "factory" farms are raised in extremely small cages (usually in their own feces) and rarely see the light of day. Furthermore, they are fed a constant supply of antibiotics and growth hormones to speed growth, keep them alive, and fend off disease (Chek 2004). This fact alone should encourage you to spend the extra money on free-range organic chicken and pork.

Understandably, the quality of an egg can be only as good as the quality of the chicken that lays it, so it is crucial to buy and eat only organic eggs. A chicken that has lived a natural life produces eggs that are extremely high in omega-3 fats—one of the healthiest types of fat for humans. As a result, the whole egg is one of the healthiest, well-balanced natural foods for humans to consume.

Many people have developed a fear of eating whole eggs because of the cholesterol in the yolk. But the truth is cholesterol is necessary for our bodies to function. However, whole eggs from commercially raised chickens are bad for us; they are high in omega-6 fats, which cause inflammation in the body and increase the risk of heart disease.

The Value of Going Organic

As explained in **Step 3: Choose the Best Foods,** anything that is toxic to the body overwhelms the liver, and an overwhelmed liver becomes clogged, which makes losing weight difficult. Pesticide residues not only clog the liver but also build up on the intestinal wall, inhibiting the absorption and digestion of nutrients from the food you eat.

Some people ask whether organic food is worth the money. To me, this question is equivalent to, "Is your health worth the money?" The most common complaint or concern about "going organic" is the expense.

Organic food is more expensive for several reasons. On average, organic farmers have lower yields and higher production costs than conventional farmers because they don't use herbicides; some crops are weeded by hand, which is labor-intensive. Also, organic farmers don't receive the many agricultural subsidies and other perks available to conventional farmers. You must weigh the extra cost in the short term with the long-term health benefits of sparing your body from all the chemicals. Consider our society's current state of health: The more chemicals and toxins we are exposed to, the worse our health becomes.

Consider this issue: If your doctor told you that you had a disease that required you to pay for special medical treatment to feel good every day, would you do it? I can confidently tell you that you can do something to protect your future health, prevent illness, and lose weight at the same time: spend the extra money on organic foods. You may find that when you spend less on packaged foods, the additional amount spent on organic produce and meats won't increase your overall grocery bill significantly. In addition, you will find that organic vegetables and fruits actually taste better than conventionally farmed ones.

Simply put, purchasing organic foods is an investment in your health.

With all of that being said, I understand that sometimes finding or even affording organic food may be a bit of a challenge for some. I know, because I personally experienced this. When I first discovered that organic foods would be better for my health, I was on a very tight budget (actually, I still adhere to a tight family budget and must also apply the ideas and strategies I am sharing below).

Lucky for you and me, the principles of Beyond Diet will still be effective and result in good weight loss and health results without going completely organic. You can implement this principle slowly, as your lifestyle and budget allows.

Here is how I mastered the art of "going organic on a budget":

1. I stopped buying processed "non foods." Most protein shakes, "health" bars, and processed foods are actually pretty expensive and when you completely eliminate them from your grocery list, you will save hundreds of dollars. Take a good look at the price of sugar cereals, packaged cookies and cakes, and frozen TV dinners. You will see how the prices of these foods quickly add up. That same amount of money can be better spent on a week's worth of organic produce.

2. When I started eating reasonable portions, the food was not that

expensive. When I really took a look at how much I was eating and how much I was supposed to be eating, I was eating almost double what a reasonable, healthy portion would be for me. When I started eating the correct portions for my weight and my goals, I began eating less but still feeling satisfied. Eating less meant spending less!

3. I sought out the local farmer's markets. The prices were so much better, and I always got fresh food in season. If there was a particular fruit that was extremely expensive during that time, I would choose a different fruit. If the berries happen to be expensive during that season, go for the apples, pears, or bananas instead. Variety is good anyway, so choose the fruits and veggies without the expensive prices.

4. I transitioned my kitchen and my whole house slowly. I probably did not have a completely organic kitchen until 3 years after I began. Not ideal, but I did the best I could. Rome wasn't built in a day, and neither was my organic palace. Do the best you can—start with a few items and go from there.

5. Buy organic foods "selectively." The following foods have been shown to have the highest levels of pesticide residue, so they should be purchased organic whenever available:

Fruits	Vegetables
1. Peaches	1. Spinach
2. Apples	2. Bell Peppers
3. Strawberries	3. Celery
4. Nectarines	4. Potatoes
5. Pears	5. Hot Peppers
6. Cherries	
7. Raspberries	
8. Imported Grapes	

These foods tend to be lower in pesticide levels so can be purchased conventional if necessary:

Fruits	Vegetables
1. Pineapples	1. Cauliflower
2. Plantains	2. Brussels Sprouts
3. Mangoes	3. Asparagus
4. Bananas	4. Radishes
5. Watermelon	5. Broccoli
6. Plums	6. Onions
7. Kiwi Fruit	7. Okra
8. Blueberries	8. Cabbage
9. Papaya	9. Eggplant
10. Grapefruit	
11. Avocado	

Frequently Asked Questions

I know Organic food is better, but it's just so expensive, what should I do?

Start by first checking the prices on some of the expensive processed foods you may be buying. For example, many unhealthy cereals today are quite pricey.

Next begin by buying the organic foods that are the most important (meats and poultry). Always look for animal products (meats, poultry, and dairy) that have no added antibiotics and growth hormones. Ingesting meats that have been injected with these harmful substances is equivalent to eating the hormones and antibiotics themselves. Very dangerous!

Then move on to those vegetables that do not have a protective skin (spinach, celery, berries)

Action Steps

- Begin by buying organic poultry, meat, and eggs. Most supermarkets now carry organic meats, poultry and eggs. If organic products are unavailable or difficult to obtain, then the next best choice is free-range, antibiotic- and hormone-free poultry, meat, and eggs. This way, even if the animals were not fed organic feed, at least they did not receive antibiotics and hormones.

- After you have made a regular practice of buying organic (or free-range, antibiotic- and hormone-free) meat, poultry, and eggs, start buying organic produce. Begin with the produce that tends to have the highest pesticide residues as listed above.

- Remember that your success on Beyond Diet is not dependent on going completely "organic." You can still see incredible weight loss results by transitioning to organic foods slowly. Just the single step of incorporating more fruits and vegetables and natural proteins into your meal plans is a great step in the right direction towards your weight loss goals.

7: Fats

Because fat is so important for so many bodily functions, you must consume an adequate amount of fat each day. Unfortunately, our society has developed a fear of fat. In turn, many companies have produced fat-free or low-fat products that contain high amounts of sugar or high-fructose corn syrup, both of which increase hunger and cravings for sugary foods.

Because fats are an essential part of any meal plan, it is important to recognize them as good or bad. In this chapter, you'll learn how to tell the difference.

Fats to Avoid

All fats are not created equal. The most detrimental fats are hydrogenated ones called trans-fatty acids (also called TFAs or "trans fats")—most commonly listed as hydrogenated oils or partially hydrogenated oils on food labels—and should be avoided in your diet.

Hydrogenation is a chemical hardening method commonly used to create fats that are shelf-stable and have a higher melting point than their source material. To hydrogenate a liquid vegetable oil, the oil is first washed, bleached, and deodorized and then heated to a high temperature along with a metal catalyst (nickel, zinc, or copper). Next, hydrogen gas is bubbled through the mixture. Partial hydrogenation results in a product that is semisolid at room temperature (like margarine or a salad dressing oil that doesn't separate), and full hydrogenation results in a product that is solid at room temperature (like Crisco shortening). Regardless of the ultimate result, hydrogenation completely alters the liquid oil's molecular structure so that it no longer resembles a natural fat; in fact, it becomes an unhealthy trans fat. Because the body does not recognize the transformed molecule as a natural fat, it cannot process it and treats it as a toxin.

The molecular structure of a trans-fatty acid is closer to that of plastic than to that of a normal fatty acid (Chek 2004). Still, many processed foods—even some considered to be healthy—are laden with trans fats. Food manufacturers use hydrogenated oils because they have a long shelf life and are cheaper to use than the real thing, but research has shown that these fats are detrimental to your health.

Trans fats can raise levels of low-density lipoproteins (LDLs, commonly known as "bad cholesterol") and lead to clogged arteries, elevated cholesterol levels, heart disease, type 2 diabetes, and even cancer (Mercola with Droege 2003). The body has no use for trans fats and stores them in fat cells and arteries. Consuming trans fats actually causes fat cravings; these cravings continue until the body receives the essential fatty acids (EFAs)—the good fats—that it needs.

Good Fats

Good fats are derived from healthy food sources. Consuming adequate amounts of the ideal fats for your metabolism type—naturally occurring in your food, used in cooking, or taken as supplements—will fulfill your daily nutritional needs and keep you from getting hungry.

Essential Fatty Acids

The human body cannot survive without some fats—specifically, EFAs. EFAs are necessary for the healthy function of every bodily process, including:

- brain and nervous system activity,
- regulation of hormones,
- function of organs and the immune system,
- cell function, and
- digestion.

Our bodies need EFAs but cannot make them on their own; therefore, we must get them from the foods we eat. The two kinds of EFAs are omega-3 and omega-6. Foods that are high in omega-6 fats are grains; commercially raised meats; oils used in processed foods; and many commonly used cooking oils, including corn, safflower, and sunflower. Omega-3 fats are found in leafy green vegetables, oily fish (like salmon), walnuts, organic eggs, and naturally-raised meats.

The ideal ratio of omega-3 to omega-6 fats is between 1:2 and 1:4. Unfortunately, because the typical American diet is abundant in grains and cooked oils, and lacking in vegetables and healthy fish, the average omega-6 intake is high and omega-3 intake low. This ratio has been calculated in some people to be as high as 1:50! Clearly, we must make a conscious effort to reduce the amount of omega-6s and increase the amount of omega-3s that we consume to bring that ratio back toward its ideal.

Omega-3 fats are vital for the development and maintenance of the adult brain and nervous system. In *The Omega Diet,* Artemis Simopoulos and Jo Robinson (1998) describe a study in which mice fed a diet low in omega-3 fats (i.e., the most common American diet—lots of carbohydrates; packaged, processed, and fast foods; minimal fruits, vegetables, and whole foods) led to a decreased mental performance compared with mice fed a diet with adequate omega-3s.

Simopoulos and Robinson (1998) also state that many behavioral and mood disorders are associated with a lack of omega-3 or an imbalance between omega-3 and omega-6 fats in the diet. Their list of recognized disorders (Simopoulos and Robinson 1998, 16) includes but is not limited to:

- asthma,
- attention-deficit/hyperactivity disorder (ADHD),
- cancer,
- depression (even among children),
- diabetes,
- heart attack,
- insulin resistance,
- obesity, and
- stroke.

While I normally like to keep supplements to a minimum and focus more on nutrients from fresh foods, fish oil supplementation may be vital if you do not consume fresh fish on a regular basis. Also, the health of our oceans—and thus the health of the fish that live in them—is not as good as it used to be. Elevated mercury levels are increasingly found in most fresh fish sold for human consumption. Incorporate one serving of fresh fish (especially wild salmon) every week or two, but avoid fish that often have elevated levels of mercury, such as tuna, shark, and swordfish. Whatever your choices, consume at least two or three servings of omega-3 fats daily.

The Truth About Saturated Fat

Heart disease was quite rare before 1920—so rare that the electrocardiograph (which performs the test now commonly known as an electrocardiogram [ECG]), developed to diagnose coronary heart disease, was considered a waste of time and quickly rejected. Apparently, no one suffered from clogged arteries at that time. But by the mid-1950s, heart disease was the leading cause of death among Americans. Today, heart disease causes at least 40% of all deaths in the United States each year.

In "The Skinny on Fats" (2001), the well-known nutritional expert Sally Fallon states that

> "If, as we have been told, heart disease results from the consumption of saturated fats, one would expect to find a corresponding increase in animal fat in the American diet over the same amount of time as the increase in heart disease. Actually, the converse is true. During the sixty-year period from 1910–1970, the proportion of traditional animal fat in the American diet declined from 83 percent to 62 percent, and butter consumption plummeted from eighteen pounds [eight kilograms] per person each year to four pounds [about two kilograms]. During the past eighty years, the consumption of dietary cholesterol intake has increased only one percent."

If saturated fat consumption actually decreased, then what increased? During the same period, the average intake of dietary vegetable oils (in the form of margarine, shortening, and refined oils) increased by about 400%, and the consumption of sugar and processed foods increased by about 60% (Fallon 2001).

Given this data, saturated fats apparently have been falsely accused; they are not the cause of modern disease. Unfortunately, people have been led to believe otherwise, so they try to avoid any food that contains high levels of saturated fat.

Coconut oil contains primarily saturated fat but no trans fat. It is rich in lauric acid, which is known for its antiviral, antibacterial, and antifungal properties. Some medical doctors now recommend coconut oil as a healthy food oil. In the informative online newsletter *Doctor House Call*, Al Sears, M.D. (2007), states, "The saturated fat found in coconut oil is a unique fat that helps prevent heart disease, helps to build up the immune system, and does not turn into fat in your body. In fact, it helps to speed up your metabolism … helping you to burn fat and increase your energy!" And Joseph Mercola, D.O. (2003), claims, "Coconut oil is truly the healthiest oil you can consume" and urges readers to try virgin coconut oil and "experience the health benefits for yourself."

The saturated fat in coconut oil (as well as in palm kernel oil) is of the medium-chain fatty acid (MCFA) variety. The body digests MCFAs more easily and uses them differently than other fats. MCFAs are sent directly to the liver, where they are immediately converted into energy. In other words, the body uses the fat to make energy rather than store it (Fife 2001).

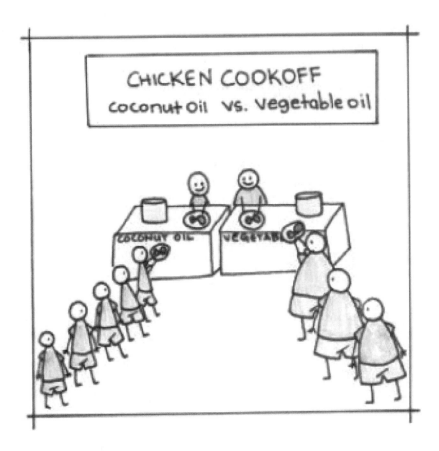

Cooking with Fats

Different types of fats respond differently to heat. Each fat has a smoke point—that is, the temperature at which it begins to smoke, become discolored, and decompose (i.e., when the fatty acid content is damaged). To avoid turning a fat rancid and unhealthy, never heat it to its smoke point. Refer to the **Cooking with Fats** chart to choose the best fat for each type of cooking.

In general, the two best fats to use for cooking are unrefined coconut oil (for very high heat) and raw organic butter (for medium-high heat; it should not turn brown during cooking). Because they contain high levels of saturated fat, they stay chemically stable up to 375°F. Oils that are low in saturated fat and high in monounsaturated fat, such as olive oil, are best consumed raw (e.g., on salads and vegetables) or used for light sautéing over medium heat.

Although coconut oil provides a significant amount of fat and calories, it has been proven to increase the body's metabolic rate, making it easier to lose weight. This program does not limit the amount that you can use each day. This is not to say that you should eat spoonful after spoonful all day long; a reasonable amount would be 1–2 tsp [5-10 mL] three times per day for cooking. I have never had a client not lose weight because of using too much coconut oil.

I know you're going to find it difficult to believe, but butter—at least the raw organic kind—is one of the healthiest whole foods you can include in your diet. Yes, butter contains high levels of saturated fat; but remember, saturated fat is not the culprit behind weight gain and high rates of disease. Trans fats (hydrogenated oils), sugars, and processed grains are the bad guys. Like coconut oil, butter is high in lauric acid, which the body uses for energy.

Extra-virgin olive oil is another healthy oil. It is rich in antioxidants, and 1 or 2 teaspoons [5-10 mL] go a long way (on a salad or in a sauté). When buying olive oil, look for oil that is cloudy (indicating that it has not been filtered) and has a golden yellow color (which means that it was made from fully ripened olives). Extra virgin is best. And, of course, it should be organic.

Action Steps

- Clean out your cupboards of all foods and snacks that contain hydrogenated or partially hydrogenated oil. You will find it in more packaged foods than you think, including many crackers, chips, pretzels, cookies, cereal bars, ready-to-eat cereals, microwave popcorn, and low-fat and fat-free snacks.

- Change your mind-set to no longer associate snacking with chips, crackers, and popcorn. Perfect snacks can be a smaller version of a real meal, such as a hard-boiled egg, a few pieces of chicken with vegetables, chopped vegetables, fruit, nuts, or nut butters. Fresh food is always the best food.

- Only use quality fats for cooking: coconut oil, butter (raw organic), and olive oil (unfiltered, organic, extra virgin). Brands and sources are listed in the **Food Shopping Guide**, which can be accessed on BeyondDiet.com at: http://www.beyonddiet.com/Members/Categories/Shopping-List. Avoid margarine and shortening, which are hydrogenated vegetable oil.

- Consume at least two to three servings daily of good-quality omega-3 fats from fish oil, seeds (especially flaxseed), avocados, and nuts (raw organic), especially walnuts.

- Avoid roasted nuts. The roasting process causes the fats and oils to go rancid, and rancid oils increase free-radical damage in the body. (Free radicals accelerate aging.) Some people find they digest nuts best when soaked overnight in filtered water and sea salt then dried in the oven the next day at a low temperature (no more than 150 degrees).

Action Steps (Cont.)

- Snack on organic nut butters. Most stores carry peanut, almond, cashew, and macadamia nut butters. The ingredient list should contain one kind of nut, salt, and nothing else. Most peanut butters contain roasted peanuts, so read labels carefully.

- Incorporate whole organic eggs into your diet, with breakfast or as a snack.

- When cooking with fat, add the fat to a cold pan and increase heat gradually.

- Serve flaxseed oil, cod liver oil, or fish oil straight from the bottle, on salads, or on cooked vegetables. Refrigerate these oils to avoid rancidity.

- If you find it difficult to incorporate foods rich in omega-3 fats into your meal plan, take an omega-3 supplement daily. A great option is BioTrust OmegaKrill 5X: http://go.beyonddiet.com/biotrustomegakrill

8: Dairy

The subject of cow's milk dairy could fill a whole book itself. As a society, we have grown up with the idea that milk and cheese should be staples in the American diet, primarily for the calcium they purportedly provide. What researchers now know is that the quality of our milk supply has drastically changed over the past century, thus changing the daily recommended requirements for dairy from three to none. Also, many Americans now suffer from lactose intolerance and thus resort to nondairy alternatives, which often end up causing problems worse than the dairy itself.

In this chapter, I will explain the changes in our dairy supply and the possible implications of conventional dairy consumption.

The Raw Alternative

My theories and beliefs about dairy products (i.e., milk, yogurt, and cheese) surprise many people. I believe that the only dairy products humans should consume are unpasteurized and unhomogenized, from free-roaming grass-fed cattle. Although some people fear becoming ill from raw dairy, thousands of people in this country (my family included) consume it, and not only are we not becoming sick from it, we're healthier than people who consume pasteurized dairy products.

Raw dairy can be difficult to obtain. You may have to find a raw dairy co-op that would allow you to buy a share in the ownership of a cow; in most states, the law allows the consumption of raw milk from a cow that you own, just not the sale of that milk to the public (for sources, see the **Food Shopping Guide**, located online at http://www.beyonddiet.com/Members/Categories/Shopping-List).

From an economic perspective, raw milk is more costly to produce (because of the extra care given to the cows), and consumers may not be willing to pay the higher price for raw milk when cheap pasteurized milk is available. This difference is equivalent to spending more money on organic food, which may be more costly to produce but is significantly more healthy than conventionally grown food.

Conventional Milk Processing

Pasteurization

In the early 1900s, milk pasteurization began for fear of tuberculosis, botulism, and a myriad of other diseases being spread through the milk supply. Whereas this concern may have been legitimate at that time, many health professionals were (and still are) against pasteurization. For example, in *The Medical Mafia* (1995), Ghislaine Lanctôt points out that the bacteria that cause typhoid and tuberculosis are not killed by the temperatures used in pasteurization (because they are not high enough), and a good number of salmonella poisoning epidemics have been traced to pasteurized milk. In fact, all of the many incidents of *Salmonella*-contaminated milk in recent decades occurred in pasteurized milk. One Illinois outbreak of salmonella poisoning in 1985 sickened 14,000 people and resulted in at least one death (Fallon 2001).

Because it contains bacteria that protect it from pathogens, unpasteurized milk probably does not cause illness; unfortunately, it is pasteurization that kills off this beneficial bacteria. Whereas raw milk eventually turns to buttermilk or sour cream, pasteurized milk can cause serious illness when it has gone bad.

Modern milking, packaging, and distributing methods are more sanitary than they were when pasteurization was first thought to be necessary. In my opinion, pasteurization is unnecessary and harms the milk. Lanctôt (1995) states that pasteurization destroys milk's intrinsic germicidal properties as well as its healthy enzymes (most of which are necessary for proper digestion). She goes on to state that 50% of pasteurized milk's calcium is unusable—the body cannot assimilate it. It is no wonder that the United States, rated highest in the amount of milk consumed, has a higher incidence of osteoporosis than any other country.

Many people experience extreme digestive discomfort (lactose intolerance) after consuming pasteurized dairy, which also may be laden with chemicals (added to suppress odor and restore taste) and synthetic vitamin D2 (toxic and linked to heart disease) or D3 (which is difficult to absorb) (Fallon 2001). In raw milk and raw milk products, the enzymes that aid in digestion are intact—as are the vitamins (Chek 2004). Most people who have experienced sensitivity to pasteurized dairy can tolerate raw milk.

Homogenization

Homogenization is a process whereby milk is passed through a fine filter that makes the fat molecules smaller. It enables the fat molecules to bypass digestion, increases the chances of incomplete protein digestion in the small intestine, and allows some of the milk proteins to be absorbed into the bloodstream intact, which can sensitize the immune system and lead to milk allergy and intolerance (Chek 2004).

Growth Hormone and Antibiotics

Another problem with commercially produced dairy is that cows are commonly injected with growth hormones to increase milk production. Normally, a cow produces milk for about 12 weeks after giving birth. It's a strain on her organs to produce milk that quickly. During this time, she loses weight, is infertile, and is highly susceptible to diseases such as mastitis (i.e., inflammation of the udder). By injecting a cow with recombinant bovine growth hormone (rBGH), a farmer can extend milk production for another 8–12 weeks—putting the cow under additional stress to produce milk for this extended period (Chek 2004).

The administration of rBGH also increases a cow's risk of infection by 80%. If a cow gets mastitis yet is forced to continue to produce milk, pus from the udder may end up in the milk supply. If the farmer gives the cow antibiotics to treat the infection, then those antibiotics also end up in the milk.

You may wonder why the U.S. Food and Drug Administration (U.S. FDA) would approve such a horrible practice as administering rBGH to dairy cows. The FDA states, "There is no difference between milk from treated and untreated cows" (Chek 2004, 67), but the minimal research that has been done was performed by the company that produces rBGH. Of course that company would be reluctant to release any information that may be damaging to it or its product. Chek (2004) mentions one specific study conducted by this same company. He explains that all of the animals treated with rBGH got cancer—even those that ingested it orally. This study was reviewed by employees who had previously worked for the rBGH company but were working for the FDA at the time the study was conducted.

The practices of pasteurization, homogenization, and rBGH administration in the United States will continue because the dairy industry has become a big money-making business. Many farmers are not willing to spend the time, effort, or money to raise cows naturally and ensure that they roam free and eat healthy clean grass. Because the dairy industry attempts to produce as much milk as possible (to make as much profit as possible), the cows become sick and toxic, in turn necessitating the pasteurization of their milk—purportedly to protect the health of consumers.

Yogurt

What about yogurt? Yogurt can be one of the healthiest foods if it contains live cultures of *acidophilus* and *Bifidus*, which are "good" bacteria—beneficial to the colon—in large amounts. These friendly bacteria are necessary in order to produce several vitamins and for healthy digestive function. The presence of these friendly bacteria also helps in the prevention and treatment of yeast infections.

Many people who are lactose-intolerant (cannot digest milk) can consume yogurt with no negative effects. Yogurt is easier to digest than milk because the live cultures create lactase, the enzyme that lactose-intolerant people lack.

However, as with other foods, yogurt can only be as healthy as its source, and added ingredients can change it from good to bad. When purchasing yogurt, always choose an organic brand, which will be free of antibiotics and rBGH. Also, pay close attention to the sugar content. Plain yogurt will have the lowest sugar content, and fruit-added or sweetened yogurt will have the greatest amounts. Most yogurts today contain more sugar and flavorings than candy does!

Organic yogurt can be included as a carbohydrate choice. Always look for the plain varieties and ensure that it does not contain added sugar (make sure to read the ingredients for any word ending in –ose). Six ounces [168 g] of organic plain yogurt is equal to 1 carbohydrate serving. Organic Greek yogurt can also be included, but this will count as a protein choice. Two ounces [50 g] of organic Greek yogurt = 1 protein serving.

Frequently Asked Questions

How will I get enough calcium if I greatly reduce my dairy intake? Will that increase my risk for osteoporosis?

I strongly suggest most people give up dairy and dairy products. As a result, people often wonder "Where will I get my calcium from?" Yes, calcium is vital for many functions in the body, but the amount the body actually needs and can absorb is much less than most people think. The worry that a deficiency in calcium will result when excluding dairy products is completely unnecessary.

The fact is that all leafy, green vegetables and grasses are inherently high in calcium (as well as iron, magnesium, Vitamin C, and many of the B vitamins) as are celery, cauliflower, okra, onions, green beans, avocado, black beans, chickpeas, almonds, hazelnuts, and sesame seeds. You can get plenty of calcium by adding in servings of the above foods. Take into consideration that most cows only eat grass and their bodies are naturally very high in calcium. That in itself tells us a lot.

It is also important to evaluate how much calcium is really necessary to keep your bones strong and free of osteoporosis. To do so, you must understand that one of the functions calcium has in the body is to help neutralize the acid created by eating acid forming foods like sugar, coffee, soda and artificial sweeteners. If many of these acid forming, calcium robbing foods are eliminated, there will be more available calcium to create and maintain strong bones and a healthy body.

Where does cheese fit into my meal plan?

Cheese should always be organic and preferably raw. One ounce [28 g] of raw organic cheese is equal to one fat serving. Cheese does not contain enough protein by itself to be a protein choice.

What happens to milk when you heat it?

The temperatures at which we heat milk over the stove are not as high as those temperatures used in pasteurization. To ensure not to denature milk and its beneficial enzymes when heating, use a low temperature and heat slowly.

Can I use Almond Milk or Rice Milk?

Almond Milk and/or Rice Milk may be good alternatives for some when dairy and soy milk are no longer an option. Unfortunately, many brands of Almond Milk and Rice Milk contain some form of unhealthy oil (like safflower oil) and high amounts of sugar. If you can find a brand that does not add sugar or oil, it is ok. In many cases, people may choose to make their own Almond Milk with the following recipe:

Ingredients
1 cup raw almonds, soaked 4 or more hours
3-6 cups water
1 Tbsp Stevia
A pinch of sea salt

Directions – Blend everything together until the texture is creamy. You can vary the amount depending on your taste. Add more water and strain if you like it thin, or add less water to get a thicker, "whipped cream" consistency. Store in a lidded jar in the fridge.

Action Steps

- If you consume dairy on a regular basis, try to buy raw (unpasteurized) certified organic products.

- If you can't obtain raw dairy products, purchase the next best thing: certified organic. Although the milk may be pasteurized, homogenized, or both, it won't contain antibiotics, hormones, or pesticide residues.

- If you can't obtain or afford raw or organic dairy products, avoid dairy altogether. Most of the calcium in dairy is not absorbed by the body anyway, so dairy is not necessary for a healthy diet. Obtain calcium from other sources, such as leafy green vegetables, broccoli, sardines (with bones), and salmon.

9: Soy

Because I recommend eliminating cow's milk from the diet, most people ask me how to replace it. Most often, they ask about soy milk.

Unfortunately, many people have been led to believe that soy and soy products are wonderfoods, but I believe that soy milk is much worse than conventional cow's milk. A lot of the "health" claims made by the soy industry are simply marketing tactics to make us spend money on soy products. The little soybean is big business; retail sales increased from $0.852 billion to $3.2 billion from 1992 to 2002. To accomplish this feat, the soy industry has had to convince a lot of people that soy is good and suppress a lot of evidence to the contrary. This truth has come to anger the many vegetarians who have long used soy as a meat replacement and now suffer from a long list of reproductive difficulties or hypothyroidism (Daniel 2005). In this chapter, I will explain why to avoid soy.

History

The soybean is an oil-rich Asian legume (bean) that grows in fuzzy green pods. Traditionally, soybean plants were grown in Asia as green manure—a crop to be plowed under to enrich the soil between crop plantings. The Chinese found that soy consumption led to digestive discomfort, bloating, and gas. Not until they came up with fermentation methods did soy begin to be used as a food for humans.

Fermented soy products such as miso, tempeh, natto, shoyu (soy sauce), and tamari are fine to eat occasionally; fermentation deactivates some of the anti-nutrients in soy that cause digestive distress and mineral loss in bones. However, the majority of soy products sold in the United States are unfermented, so the naturally occurring toxins are intact. Unfermented soy products also are processed in a way that makes their proteins impure and increases the amount of carcinogens (Daniel 2005).

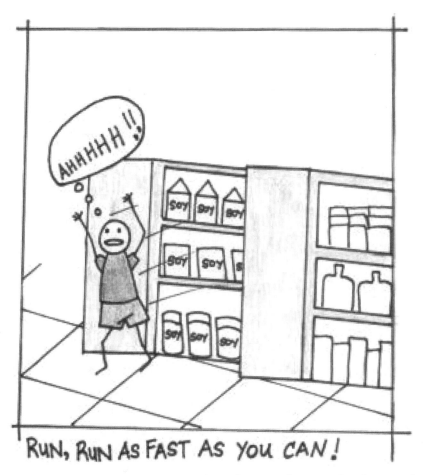

RUN, RUN AS FAST AS YOU CAN!

Some people argue that since Asians have been eating soy for thousands of years and have an incidence of cancer far lower than Americans, small amounts of natural fermented soy in the average Asian diet (9.3–36 grams [2–4 teaspoons] of soy per day as a condiment) may well have a protective effect. Unfortunately, Americans have taken this information and applied it incorrectly to highly processed, unfermented, low-quality soy products like tofu (a single cup of which weighs 252 grams). Many Americans eat several cups of soy products daily.

Soyfoods

In the West, the soybean has been used mostly as soybean oil, which is found in most products labeled as vegetable oil, margarine, or shortening. The soy protein left over from soy oil extraction originally was fed exclusively to animals—poultry and, more recently, farmed fish. The problem is that animals can consume only so much soy before developing serious reproductive and other health problems. As a result, the soy industry started marketing these by-products of soybean oil production to people.

A product of the industrial revolution, soy gave food technologists an opportunity to develop cheap meat substitutes. The most unhealthy modern soyfood products are manufactured using high-tech processes. They include ready-made foods such as soy sausages, soy burgers, chicken-like soy patties, packaged soy milk, protein powders, energy bars, veggie burgers, low-carbohydrate pastas, and chilis, as well as countless foods containing soy protein isolate, soy protein concentrate, and texturized vegetable protein.

Soy Isoflavones

Hormonal Effects

Just about all soy products on the market contain the phytoestrogens (plant-derived estrogens) known as isoflavones (Daniel 2005). Soy isoflavones have been shown to decrease the testosterone levels of rats, monkeys, and other animals, including humans.

In adults, soy consumption may disrupt normal hormone levels, effecting the reproductive system in women (resulting in heavier menstrual flow, increased cramping, and infertility) and decreasing testosterone levels in men (which decreases libido and lowers sperm count). In fact, a Japanese old wives' tale says that women punish straying husbands by feeding them a lot of tofu!

The effects of soy are no laughing matter, especially when it comes to the health and development of infants who are fed soy formula. Infants are extremely susceptible to the effects of soy because formula constitutes most, if not all, of their diets. Figures from the Swiss Federal Health Service indicate that, on a daily basis, an infant who is fed soy formula receives an amount of estrogen equivalent to that found in three to five birth control pills (Daniel 2005)! That's a lot of estrogen for anyone, but this amount is especially dangerous for infants whose development requires the right hormones in the right place at the right time. In boys, the onset of puberty may be delayed, and pediatricians are increasingly reporting cases of emasculated boys who reach puberty with breasts and tiny penises (Daniel 2005). In girls, the onset of puberty may be accelerated, and reproductive problems may occur in adulthood.

Thyroid Effects

Soy isoflavones damage more than the reproductive system in adults and children. People who consume high amounts of soy protein each day (e.g., in soy milk and in high-protein energy bars, which contain soy isolates—the most concentrated source of soy, still containing its isoflavones and phytoestrogens) often complain of fatigue, low energy, depression, hair loss, poor skin, weight gain, and diminished sex drive—all symptoms of low thyroid function (Daniel 2005). When tested for hypothyroidism, these people almost always test positive.

Action Steps

- Discard everything in your cupboards that contains soy protein isolate, soy protein concentrate, texturized vegetable protein, or soy (or soybean) oil. Possible products include many packaged energy bars, crackers, veggie burgers, and vegetarian look-alike products.

- If you have been consuming soy for a long time, get your thyroid function checked. If you suffer from hypothyroidism, then eliminating soy from your diet may have a positive effect on your condition.

10: Grains

For several million years, humans survived on a diet of animals and plants. As hunter–gatherers, they ate whatever they could find. With the introduction of new farming practices 10,000 years ago, humans began eating sugar and starch (in the form of grains and potatoes).

Although 10,000 years sounds like a long time, it's really only a fraction of a second in evolutionary terms, and the human body and digestive system have not evolved to process and digest high amounts of carbohydrates from starch- and sugar-rich diets. Genetically speaking, humans still have the bodies of cavemen.

Carbohydrates

Most Americans eat far too many carbohydrates—in the form of bread, cereal, pasta, corn (a grain, not a vegetable), rice, potatoes, and processed cakes and snacks—with severe consequences to their health. Making matters worse, most of these carbohydrates are consumed in the form of processed foods. After 130 years of consuming highly processed grains in the form of breads, pastries, and cereals, chronic diseases such as heart disease, elevated cholesterol, and obesity are rampant among most industrialized nations.

I do not suggest that everyone should follow a low-carbohydrate diet; everyone needs a certain amount of carbohydrates. What most people haven't realized is that the body's storage capacity for carbohydrates is quite limited, and any excess is stored as fat. Therefore, it is important to remember that vegetables and fruits also contain carbohydrates and to make the appropriate carbohydrate choices for your metabolism type. For example, the ideal foods for a Protein Type may include more above-ground vegetables and few fruits, whereas a Carb Type can tolerate starchier root vegetables and grains.

Any meal or snack high in carbohydrates generates a rapid rise in blood glucose (sugar). To compensate for this increase, the pancreas secretes insulin into the bloodstream, which lowers the glucose. Insulin, though, is essentially a hormone that stores excess carbohydrate calories (as fat in the thighs, abdomen, and buttocks) in case of famine. Even worse, high insulin levels suppress two other important hormones: glucagon and human growth hormone, which regulate the burning of fat and promote muscle development, respectively. So, the insulin from excess carbohydrates promotes fat, then inhibits the body's ability to lose that fat.

The key to successful weight loss is to first find the right quantity of carbohydrates that provide enough fuel and energy for the day (but not so many that we end up storing most of it as fat), then consume the right kind of carbohydrates to feel good and satiated after a meal.

Bread

Probably the most consumed and most popular of all carbohydrates among Americans is bread. Americans consume far too much bread, and the negative effects of its consumption are manifest in poor health and excess weight. Americans also consume the wrong kinds of bread.

The only bread allowed on this program is Food for Life brand's Ezekiel 4:9 organic sprouted whole grain (SWG) products. The process of sprouting changes a grain's composition in numerous ways to make it more beneficial as a food. It increases the content of vitamins (e.g., C, B2, B5, and B6) and beta carotene dramatically, up to eightfold. Even more important—especially considering how many people suffer from indigestion—it breaks down phytic acid (a mineral blocker). Present in the bran of all grains and the coatings of nuts and seeds, phytic acid inhibits the body's absorption of calcium, magnesium, iron, copper, and zinc and can neutralize digestive enzymes, resulting in digestive disorders. Sprouting breaks down the complex sugars responsible for intestinal gas and transforms a portion of the starch into sugar. It also inactivates aflatoxins, which are toxins produced by fungus and potent carcinogens often found in grains (Chek 2004).

The whole wheat bread that the American public has been led to believe is healthy contains processed wheat, which is deficient in nutrients. Hence the extremely high prevalence among Americans of digestive disorders such as irritable bowel syndrome and constipation. Chronic constipation can lead to many potentially dangerous health disorders and also can make losing weight quite difficult. Simply replacing bread with SWG bread can radically improve your digestion and your ability to lose weight.

Note that if you are intolerant of gluten or wheat, then you also will be intolerant of Ezekiel 4:9 organic sprouted whole grain bread. Even though sprouted grains are healthy foods for most people, the Ezekiel 4:9 ingredients include wheat and other grains that contain gluten.

Glycemic Index

Because the body converts different types of carbohydrates into sugar at different rates, the glycemic index (GI) was established to indicate how quickly a food affects blood sugar levels. Foods that have a high GI cause a rapid increase in blood glucose levels, thus a rapid release of insulin, which is exactly what you don't want when trying to lose weight and maintain good health. Foods that have a low GI cause a slow increase in blood glucose levels and a slow and controlled insulin release.

As explained earlier, insulin is a fat-storing hormone, so the more you have coursing through your bloodstream, the more likely you are to gain weight. Also, high-GI foods tend to leave you feeling hungry and craving more, whereas low-GI foods make you feel satiated and free from cravings. Refer to the **Glycemic Index** chart to learn the GI of each carbohydrate.

Weight loss will be much easier if you choose low-GI carbohydrates: vegetables and some (not all) fruits. Certain types of grains and beans also have a low GI. I highly recommend that you stay away from high-GI foods when weight loss and overall health are your goals.

Gluten Intolerance

Many people cannot digest gluten—a protein found in wheat and some other grains that forms the structure of bread dough—and suffer from a mild to severe gluten intolerance. Possible symptoms of gluten intolerance include

- abdominal pain and cramping,

- bloating and flatulence,

- bone and joint pain,

- chronic diarrhea,

- emotional disturbances such as anxiety and depression,

- fatigue (especially after eating gluten-containing foods),

- infertility,

- painful skin rash, and

- weight gain or the inability to lose weight.

If you suspect that you may be intolerant to gluten, I encourage you to eliminate gluten from your diet for at least 4–6 weeks to determine whether your symptoms are alleviated. Some **gluten-containing foods** and ingredients to avoid include the following:

- barley

- beer

- cold cereals (some—read ingredient lists)

- couscous

- hydrolyzed vegetable protein

- oats

- pasta

- rye

- semolina

- soy sauce

- spelt

- starch and vegetable starch

- wheat

- wheat germ

Allowable gluten-free foods and ingredients include the following:

- amaranth

- arrowroot

- bean flours (e.g., garbanzo, sorghum)

- buckwheat

- corn

- millet

- quinoa

- rice

If you feel relief from any of the above-named symptoms after following a gluten-free diet for 4–6 weeks, then you may be able to maintain a healthy weight more easily without gluten. Because most individuals who are intolerant to gluten also are intolerant to dairy, lactose, or both, I encourage you to also eliminate dairy and dairy-containing products while you're on a gluten-free diet.

Eliminating Grains

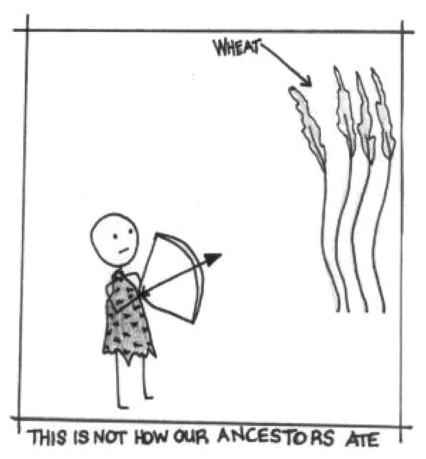

Many health experts recommend that people who suffer from chronic disease (e.g., diabetes, high blood pressure, high cholesterol, or heart disease), have struggled with obesity their whole lives, or are genetically predisposed to obesity or chronic disease completely eliminate grains from their diet. Joseph Mercola, an internationally renowned natural health physician and doctor of osteopathy, says that the major culprit behind various chronic diseases and the obesity epidemic is the overconsumption of grains and sugar. His *Total Health Program* (Mercola 2005) and *The No-Grain Diet* (Mercola with Levy 2003) teach optimal health and weight through grain elimination.

Mercola's No-Grain Diet (which also eliminates some other foods, such as dairy and beans) has been referred to as the Paleolithic Diet or the Caveman Diet because the allowed foods are those that were available to man before the discovery of grains. It is essentially how the first humans ate 2 million years ago. Some dieticians believe the Paleolithic Diet is the only diet coded in human genes—it allows only those foods that were available during our long evolution and discards those that were not.

Foods eliminated on a grain-free diet include

- all gluten and gluten-free grains (as well as bread, pasta, and noodles made from grains)

- corn and corn-based products

- dairy products

- legumes (e.g., string beans, kidney beans, lentils, peanuts, snow peas, and green peas)

- potatoes (white and sweet) and yams

- sugar

Foods allowed on a grain-free diet include

- eggs

- fruits and berries

- meat, chicken, and fish

- tree nuts (except cashews)

- vegetables (especially green vegetables)

I prescribe this way of eating to clients who have a history of diabetes, high blood pressure, high cholesterol, and heart disease or who have a long history of weight gain and difficulty losing weight. The results are truly amazing. Clients have told me that within the first week, their aches and pains went away and that they felt so much lighter and more energetic throughout the day. People suffering from digestive difficulties often feel relief in just a few days.

Frequently Asked Questions

What about Rice, wheat and grains which are very prominent in my native foods?

Rice and wheat are very high in calories and carbohydrates, even in small servings. Many people are also intolerant to wheat and this intolerance makes it very difficult for them to lose their unwanted weight. Instant rice, rice bowls, and any other rice products that have added creams, sauces or tons of sodium are not recommended, but many other types of rice (white rice, basmati rice, black rice, jasmine, wild rice... all in moderation) are ok choices and acceptable on the Beyond Diet plan.

How about brown rice?

Although many people consider brown rice a health food, it is high in phytic acid which has the ability to grab onto other important minerals in your body, like calcium, magnesium, iron and zinc. Our bodies do not have the ability to breakdown phytic acid (in brown rice) and eating it can lead to mineral deficiencies. Phytic acid also inhibits enzymes that we need to digest our foods, including pepsin, which we need to digest proteins. I highly suggest you keep your intake of brown rice low, 1-2 times per month at the most, and choose from white rice, basmati rice, black rice, jasmine rice and wild rice more often.

Keep in mind that the glycemic index of a food changes drastically when combined with other foods. So regardless of your rice choice, it is essential that you combine your rice (a carb) with a healthy protein and fat any and every time you eat it. A good example of a well proportioned meal would be 1/2 cup cooked wild rice, 4 oz bison burger, small green salad with olive oil and vinegar dressing.

Where does Rye bread fit into my carbohydrate choices?

Rye is in the same family as wheat and does still contain "gluten" which is the protein in breads that causes bloating. If you are staying away from wheat and gluten containing product, you should stay away from Rye as well.

Sprouted whole grain breads, and breads made from rice and spelt are still your best option.

Action Steps

- For all of your bread needs, consume only Food for Life's Ezekiel 4:9 organic sprouted whole grain (SWG) products (e.g., original, sesame, and cinnamon raisin loaves; rolls; English muffins; and tortillas). Use this bread to make bread crumbs for meatloaf and meatball recipes.

- Accept that breakfast and lunch do not have to include toast and sandwiches. Depending on your metabolism type, eggs, fruits, and nut butters may be great options for breakfast. Salads or vegetables with poultry, fish, or other meats may be great options for lunch.

- If you experience gastrointestinal distress (gas or bloating) while following this program, you may be gluten-intolerant. Try eliminating all gluten grains for 4–6 weeks to see whether the condition improves.

- If you continue to suffer from gastrointestinal distress after eliminating gluten grains for 4–6 weeks or if you do not lose weight after 4 weeks on this program, eliminate all grains from your diet.

11: Salt

Many people follow a low-salt diet because they have been led to believe that salt and sodium are bad and unhealthy. In this chapter I will explain why this belief may only be partially true and why salt is important in the body for several functions.

Chemically, culinary salt is NaCl—sodium chloride, made up of equal amounts sodium (Na) and chloride (Cl). "Sodium is an essential nutrient that the body cannot manufacture, yet is required for life itself. Chloride is vital for optimum health, it preserves the acid–base balance in the body, aids potassium absorption, supplies the essence of digestive stomach acid, and enhances the ability of the blood to carry carbon dioxide from respiring tissues to the lungs" (Regenerative Nutrition n.d.). But the only way to receive all of the life-sustaining benefits of salt is to consume the right kind of salt: unrefined sea salt, not processed table salt.

Salt has such a bad reputation because 99% of the world's salt research has been done on commercial table salt—the only salt that most Americans know. Some of the best scientific research on the healthy properties of unrefined sea salt are written in French, German, and Portuguese; unfortunately, few American doctors have read them. So instead of suggesting that patients use unrefined sea salt, American doctors suggest avoiding salt altogether, which can be dangerous. In many parts of France, when a person visits a physician about a heart problem or high blood pressure, the first question asked may be, "What kind of salt do you use?"

Some doctors believe that a low-salt diet can cause high blood pressure. A salt-free diet can damage heart valves and negatively affect the contractibility of the heart muscles. Biochemically, cells starve without salt.

In brief, salt

- aids in balancing blood sugar levels.
- is needed for the absorption of food particles through the intestinal tract.
- is a strong natural antihistamine.

- can help prevent muscle cramps.

- is needed to make bones strong.

- regulates and normalizes blood pressure.

- increases energy levels.

- helps regulate the metabolism.

- helps maintain proper electrolyte balance. and

- supports the immune system.

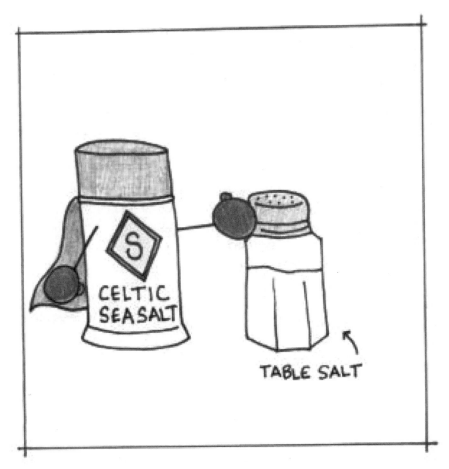

The refined white table salt typically found at the grocery store is different from unrefined sea salt, so its effects on the body are not the same. The body cannot assimilate isolated synthetic sodium chloride (from typical refined salt), which contains none of the valuable minerals and trace elements of unrefined sea salt, so the system recognizes it as a poison. Refined table salt often contains anti-caking agents, some of which are aluminum based. (Aluminum is linked with heavy metal toxicity and possibly even Alzheimer's disease.) One such example is sodium silicoaluminate, which is thought to be associated with kidney problems and mineral malabsorption. Sodium acetate, a preservative, may cause elevated blood pressure, kidney disturbances, and water retention (Chek 2004).

I recommend that you replace refined table salt with an unrefined sea salt like AztecSeaSalt™ or Celtic sea salt. AztecSeaSalt™ cannot be found in stores, but it can be purchased online at http://go.beyonddiet.com/aztecseasalt. Celtic sea salt can be found in most health food stores or purchased online at http://go.beyonddiet.com/getcelticseasalt. Unrefined sea salt is extremely healthy and has the exact opposite effect of refined salt. It provides sodium chloride in a form that the body needs to function. It offers the perfect balance of minerals, nutrients, and sodium chloride that the body needs for optimum health. Your body can recognize and absorb these essential nutrients efficiently. Over 80 trace minerals found in the naturally filtered salt water used to create unrefined sea salt give it its vital grayish color, and its slight moistness keeps the salt and minerals in a form that the body can assimilate (Regenerative Nutrition).

Even heart patients and people with high blood pressure can use Celtic sea salt (but they will receive its benefits only if they eliminate all forms of processed salt, sodium, and table salt from their diets). The heart is fed by a saline solution from the blood and lymph and requires proper amounts of sodium and potassium to function. Without salt in the diet, the heart cannot contract normally, and the valves may be damaged (Regenerative Nutrition). If you don't salt your food, add a pinch of sea salt to each liter bottle of water you drink to maintain electrolyte and energy levels.

Clearly, salt is important to optimum health. Processed table salt is what's causing so many people to suffer from health problems such as high blood pressure. Simply eating salty food is not the answer; using unrefined sea salt it. The sodium in this healthy form of salt is the actual sodium that our bodies need to function properly. As with other dietary recommendations, moderation is always essential.

Frequently Asked Questions

Is it ok to use unrefined Sea Salt even if I have high blood pressure?

Yes. Unrefined Sea Salt is safe even for those with high blood pressure. It has been found that the sodium in this healthy form of salt is the actual sodium that our bodies need to function properly. Processed table salt is what's causing so many people to suffer from health problems such as high blood pressure. I highly recommend you stay away from all refined table salt and include unrefined sea salt into your meal plans.

Unfortunately many sea salts, even most of the ones sold at Trader Joe's, are still refined.

I get all my salt from this site: http://go.beyonddiet.com/aztecseasalt

Action Steps

- Avoid all refined white table salt.

- Avoid all high-sodium packaged and canned foods.

- Use unprocessed, unrefined AztecSeaSalt™, Himalayan pink salt, Celtic sea salt, or Redmond's real salt. (Other types of sea salts may contain mercury or other toxic heavy metals.)

- Always taste food before adding salt.

12: Water

If ever there were a magic potion for weight loss, water would be it. Every good nutritional program insists that you drink a minimum of 8–10 glasses of water per day. Most people don't drink the recommended amount because they don't fully understand how important water is to maintaining good health and losing weight.

Our bodies are composed of approximately 75% water. Any variation from the natural balance causes serious disruptions in many metabolic processes that are crucial to weight loss.

- **Water helps the body metabolize stored fat.** The kidneys cannot function properly without enough water. When they are not working at full capacity, the liver must take over some of the load. The liver's function is crucial to weight loss, and if the liver has to do some of the kidneys' work, it cannot adequately do its job (metabolizing fat). As a result, the liver metabolizes less fat, more fat is stored in the body, and weight loss becomes slow or stagnates.

- **Water is crucial in ridding the body of waste.** During weight loss, the body has a lot of waste to eliminate: excess fat and stored toxins. Adequate water consumption helps the body flush out these wastes.

- **Water is a natural diuretic.** Many people retain fluid and become dependent on synthetic diuretics to lose excess water weight. Surprisingly, drinking enough water is actually the best treatment for water retention. When it doesn't get enough water, the body perceives a threat to its survival and begins to hold on to every drop of water that it can. If you give your body the amount of water that it needs, it will quickly release any retained water.

- **Water is a natural laxative.** When the body does not get enough water, it takes it from other internal sources. If the colon becomes dry, stool becomes dry and difficult to pass, resulting in constipation—possibly with gas, bloating, and painful elimination. If the body receives sufficient amounts of water, the

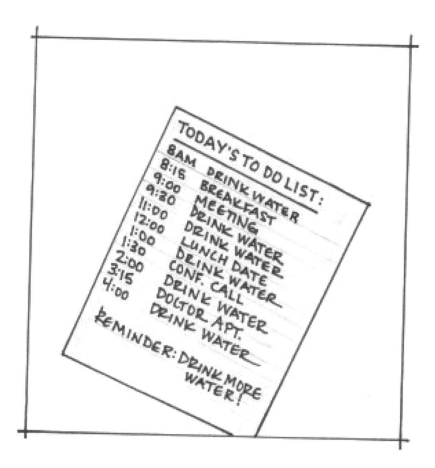

colon will be rehydrated and proper bowel function restored.

To experience significant weight loss and optimal health, it is crucial to drink a sufficient amount of water every day. By "sufficient," I mean that you should drink half your body weight (in pounds) in ounces of water each day: (body weight, in pounds/2). For example, a 200-pound person should drink 100 ounces of water. [You should drink 3 percent of your body weight (in kilos) in liters of water each day: (body weight, in kilos, x .03). For example, a 90-kilo person should drink 2.7 liters of water.]

In addition to this baseline recommendation, I suggest that you add 8 ounces [236 mL] of water for every 8 ounces [236 mL] of caffeinated beverage consumed and another 8 ounces [236 mL] if you have exercised. Also, drink water at room temperature. Cold water will sit in your stomach until it has warmed to body temperature; only then will it move to the small intestine for absorption (Chek 2004).

Many people mistake thirst for hunger because both sensations tell the brain that the body is in need of energy. As a result, a person who is dehydrated may misinterpret this feeling and end up overeating. Several studies have been done in which people were told to drink water at the first sign or feeling of hunger. In most cases, the hunger quickly passed, and subjects lost 35–40 pounds [15-20 kilos] in less than a year (Batmanghelidj 1992). If you do not drink the recommended amounts of water for your weight and experience hunger pangs during the day, then chances are your body is thirsty. Because water is a natural appetite suppressant, drink 8 ounces [236 mL] of water at the first sign of hunger and 15 minutes before the start of every meal.

Although drinking the appropriate quantity of water is essential, it is equally important to drink high-quality water. Unfortunately, no matter where you live, tap water is contaminated with heavy metals, chlorine, and waterborne toxins. I highly recommend that you filter the drinking water in your home. (Some sources are listed under **the Food Shopping Guide,** located online at http://www.beyonddiet.com/Members/Categories/Shopping-List.) If you buy bottled water, some of the best brands are Evian, Volvic, and Fiji.

Glass containers are best to keep stored water fresh and pure. Plastic containers can leach plastic by-products into the water, affecting taste and purity, especially if exposed to direct sunlight, so always keep bottled water in a dark, cool area. Never purchase water in smoky plastic containers, which leak estrogenic chemicals (which can disrupt hormone levels) and phthalates (which have been linked to asthma and allergies) into the water.

Ideally, you also should install shower filters or, better, a whole-house water filtration system. Your skin is a living organ, and absorbing high levels of metals and chlorine from your shower and bathwater can be dangerous.

Frequently Asked Questions

Can I drink green or black tea on this plan?

Yes. You can drink green, black, white, oolong and all varieties of herbal teas. Green tea has been found to contain catechins and polyphenols which act as antioxidants contributing to the prevention of cancer and accelerated aging.

While some studies have shown some teas to contribute to accelerated fat loss, the amounts are so minimal as compared to following a healthy eating and exercise regimen.

Can I still keep drinking coffee on this plan?

Yes. You may continue to drink coffee but in moderation. You should never exceed 2 – 8 oz [240 mL] cups of coffee in one day. Remember that caffeine is a drug and when you attempt to go without it, you will suffer severe withdrawal symptoms similar to any drug.

Coffee should always be organic as the conventional varieties are filled with pesticides. Pesticides are again a harmful toxin to your body. Organic Espresso is also permitted.

Drinking lots of water with coffee

The water you are drinking is only countering the dehydration you may experience from so much coffee. This still does not resolve the high amount of acidity in your body. I would slowly work towards decreasing your intake until you get to 1-2 cups. I know it's tough (I've been there) but your body will thank you :)

Decaf coffee

Most decaf coffees still contain some caffeine so they are never "caffeine-free." Also, many harmful chemicals are used in the decaffeination process so their chemical content is many times higher than regular coffee. Decaf coffee that is labeled naturally decaffeinated or Swiss water processed is much better. This still does contribute to the acidity in your body so you will want to keep your intake of decaf coffees to the same 2 cups a day maximum.

Action Steps

- Drink half of your body weight (in pounds) in ounces of water each day. Add 8 ounces of water for each 8-ounce caffeinated beverage you drink and another 8 ounces if you have exercised that day. [Drink 3 percent of your body weight (in kilos) in liters of water each day. Add 236 ml of water for each 236 ml caffeinated beverage you drink and another 236 ml of water if you have exercised that day.]

- Drink 8 ounces of water when you feel hungry.

- Drink 8 ounces of water 15 minutes before each meal.

- If you use plastic water bottles, keep them out of the sun and away from heat.

- Install filters for your drinking water and bathing water, or invest in a whole-house water filtration system. Sun Water Systems (http://go.beyonddiet.com/getaquasana) sells Aquasana brand products for kitchen, bathroom, and whole-house water filtration as well as glass bottles for water storage – best news here is that we talked with Sun Water Systems and they are willing to give Beyond Diet customers **a 10% discount** using the link above.

13: Sweeteners

I introduced some caution foods as part of the "Must Do's" for each metabolism type in the **Chapter on Metabolism Types.** However, most commercially available sweeteners are counterproductive to a healthy lifestyle for everyone.

Sugar

It is said that for every American who eats only 5 pounds [2.5 kilos] of sugar each year, another eats 295 pounds [134 kilos]. This statistic is hard to deny, because about 60% of the U.S. population is now overweight or obese (Chek 2004).

Part of my professional responsibility to you is to not downplay the serious damage that sugar can do to your body. I am passionate about communicating the harmful effects of sugar because I have seen clients and loved ones suffer from severe complications of type 2 diabetes, the onset of which was caused directly by their consumption of sugar and refined carbohydrates. Processed sugar (which is in cakes, cookies, processed cereals, and many other foods) can literally be considered a poison, which is anything that directly causes harm and can lead to a diseased state when you ingest it.

For starters, daily sugar consumption produces a continuous acidic condition in the body. The body combats an acidic condition by taking minerals from body tissues to buffer against the acidic environment and rectify the imbalance. For example, the body may absorb calcium from bones and teeth to protect the blood. As a result, bones weaken (resulting in osteoporosis) and teeth decay (resulting in cavities). Excess sugar eventually affects every organ in the body.

Sugar has been proven to be the cause of several diseases, including diabetes, cardiovascular disease, and cancer (Mercola 2005). When the liver has stored all the sugar that it can, the excess is returned to the blood in the form of fatty acids. These fatty acids are then stored as fat in the most inactive areas of the body: belly, buttocks, breasts, and thighs. When these areas become completely filled with fat, fatty acids are then distributed among active organs (heart, liver, and kidneys), increasing the risk of developing diabetes and disease in these organs.

It is well known and well documented that cancer cells can survive only in an acidic environment and will die in an alkaline (non-acidic) environment (Quillin 2005). Sugar keeps the body in an acidic state, and tumors are enormous sugar absorbers.

Sugar consumption causes a hormonal roller coaster of alternating high levels of insulin and blood sugar. These hormonal shifts can dramatically affect your attitude and your ability to concentrate during the day. Also, if you replace nutrient-dense foods with processed sugar, the chances of acquiring one of the following diseases or side-effects skyrockets (Chek 2004):

- atherosclerosis
- attention deficit disorder and attention-deficit/hyperactivity disorder
- behavior problems
- cancer
- chronic fatigue syndrome
- colon cancer
- coronary heart disease
- food intolerance
- kidney disease
- liver disease
- malnutrition
- osteoporosis
- overgrowth of yeast, especially *Candida albicans*
- tooth decay
- violent tendencies

Even if you don't consume candy or sweets outright, once you begin to read the labels of most snacks, cereals, and drinks you consume, you will notice that it doesn't take much to consume approximately 80 grams of sugar—the equivalent of 20 teaspoons [100 mL]—in a day! When reading labels, don't be thrown off by strange words like sucrose, maltose, dextrose, glucose, and the like — any word ending in -ose is a sugar. Quite often, one product will contain five or six different types of sugar. When you add up all its many forms, sugar is frequently the greatest source of total calories.

How about fruit? Fruit contains sugar, but solely in the form of fructose, whereas processed sugar (sucrose) is made up of both glucose and fructose. By itself, fructose breaks down more slowly in the body; sugar and insulin levels remain relatively constant. In contrast, sucrose is processed extremely quickly, causing a "spike" in insulin levels—rather like a power surge followed by a rapid return to baseline levels—that is stressful for the body. Fructose puts a lot less stress on the body than sucrose, and most fruits have a low GI.

The biggest mistake people make is falling for the marketing hype from juice manufacturers. They want you to think their "fresh juice" is actually good for you. If you read the package, you'll see that many such products are made "from concentrate," which could easily be translated to mean "from syrup" (Chek 2004).

Artificial Sweeteners

Some diets encourage the use of artificial sweeteners and products sweetened with them. This program does not. Consuming artificial sweeteners will keep you craving sweetness. You'll never be able to stop your carbohydrate cravings. Worse, some research indicates that artificial sweeteners create the same insulin surge as sugar (Kirsch 2005).

Artificial sweeteners signal to your taste buds, "Sweet stuff has arrived," which is translated to the brain as, "Nutrition has arrived." When the artificial sweetener reaches the small intestine, the receptors find no nutrition and send a message back to the brain, saying, "We've been tricked. There's no nutrition here." The appestat (the part of your brain that triggers satiety) therefore signals to "keep eating ... to help process all this nonfood" and keep the body functioning (Chek 2004). For this reason, many people who constantly drink diet sodas are overweight and always hungry.

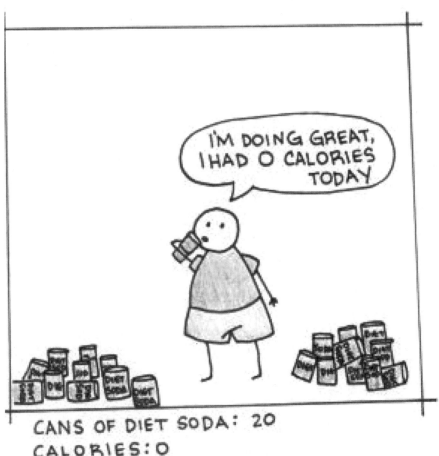

CANS OF DIET SODA: 20
CALORIES: 0
ARTIFICIAL SWEETNER: 2,620mg
NOT LOSING WEIGHT: **NOT** PRICELESS

If you eat foods that contain some form of artificial sweetener, add up how much you consume each day. Knowing now that artificial sweeteners are toxic to the liver, how overwhelmed do you think your liver is? Does it have the ability to work properly? If weight loss or avoiding sweets has always been a problem for you, then take particular notice of how much artificial sweetener you have been ingesting. It just may be the culprit. I have seen many people experience dramatic weight and health changes just by quitting diet soda!

Even if you don't intentionally use artificial sweeteners, you must read labels. Almost every diet or sugar-free product on the market has added artificial sweetener, as do some children's snacks and most flavored waters. Read ingredient lists, and avoid all products that contain saccharin (Sweet'N Low), aspartame (NutraSweet), and sucralose (Splenda).

Stevia: A Natural Alternative

Eliminating sugar and artificial sweeteners may be difficult if you are accustomed to sweet tastes. A wonderful natural alternative to both sugar and artificial sweeteners is an herb called stevia. Extraordinarily sweet (200–300 times sweeter than sugar), stevia also is almost free of calories, so it is perfect for people who are watching their weight. Unlike sugar, it doesn't trigger a rise in blood sugar, so you won't experience a sudden increase in insulin levels. Because insulin levels and blood sugar are not affected, you won't experience a burst of energy followed by fatigue and cravings.

Stevia also presents great advantages over saccharin and other artificial sweeteners—it isn't toxic, and it has been used safely for hundreds of years. It can be used to sweeten drinks and even in baking.

If you are addicted to sodas or other beverages sweetened with sugar or artificial sweeteners, try my Tea Juice recipe in the **Recipe Guide,** or view it online at http://www.beyonddiet.com/Members/Recipes/Tea-Juice_1. After only 72 hours off of sugar and sugar-containing products, your cravings will decrease drastically.

Truvia

Truvia has gotten quite a bit of attention in the media lately because it contains Stevia (a natural and healthy alternative to artificial sweeteners) but can be found at almost any local supermarket and is much cheaper than Stevia. But there is a reason why. It is not pure and contains other ingredients.

The label on the Truvia box says Erythritol, Rebiana, and Natural Flavors.

Erythritol is a natural sugar alcohol and Rebiana comes directly from the Stevia plant, but what makes me a little reluctant to use Truvia is the "Natural Flavors." When you click on the "natural flavors" link on Truvia's website to get a better explanation of what these natural flavors really are, all it says is "Natural Flavors are used to bring out the best of our natural sweetness, like pepper or salt would be used to heighten the taste of a meal." What? What does that mean? That doesn't tell me anything or indicate exactly what these natural flavors are and whether or not it could be harmful to our health.

So I don't recommend Truvia. What I recommend is natural, 100% Stevia. That is the brand I use and feel safe and confident using and recommending it.

Xylitol

Xylitol is a naturally occurring sugar in the bark of a birch tree. It is completely natural and can be used as a sweetener instead of sugar. Xylitol still does contain some calories (approximately 2.4 calories per gram compared to 4 calories per gram of sugar). Although Xylitol is a great alternative for those who wish to decrease their sugar intake, many people have a difficult time digesting Xylitol and begin to suffer from painful gas and gastrointestinal distress. Make sure to pay attention to any side effects you may be experiencing from using Xylitol.

Erythritol

Erythritol is a "sugar alcohol" that is naturally found in a wide variety of foods including mushrooms, watermelon, pears and grapes (as well as fermented foods like sake, wine and soy sauce). It has zero calories and a glycemic index of zero. And it's widely considered the "almost sugar" by health experts and pastry chefs alike. But while erythritol does a great job at mimicking the sweet taste of sugar, it behaves quite differently in the body.

First, it is slowly and incompletely absorbed from the small intestine into the blood. Then, the very small amount of erythritol that is absorbed gets converted to energy by processes that require little or no insulin. That's why erythritol won't cause a spike in blood sugar levels, which is great news for anyone who is concerned about their weight!

Honey

Honey is a wonderful and natural alternative to artificial sweetners and sugar, but it must be RAW. Raw honey is a great immune system booster, has been found to contain anti-cancer properties, helps relieve arthritis pain and assists in relieving ailments like yeast infection and athletes foot, but I cannot emphasize enough that these properties have only been found in RAW honey and not pasteurized and processed honey.

Look for honey that looks thick and cloudy and specifically says "RAW" on the label and stay away from honey that has been pasteurized or processed. As with absolutely every food, be sure to use it in moderation and pay close attention to your body's response after consuming it. I use approximately 1-2 tsps of raw honey each day in my tea or on Ezekiel bread toast with almond butter... one of my favorite pre-workout snacks.

Maple Syrup

Maple syrup, if 100% pure (no processing or removal of anything), can be a great sweetener. Maple syrup contains manganese and zinc, natural antioxidants which are good for your immune system, male reproductive systems and helps prevent damage to the heart. It has also been found to be a potent liver cleanser, ensuring that the liver performs well.

The only problem that I have seen with those who use maple syrup is that they tend to use way too much in 1 serving. One teaspoon of maple syrup can go a long way and I've even used as little as 1/2 teaspoon to sweeten drinks or hot cereals like oatmeal and quinoa. Maple syrup is not usually my first choice for a sweetener, as I tend to use stevia and raw honey the most, but it is still an acceptable choice on a healthy, fat burning meal plan.

Chocolate

Good news for chocoholics.

As a chocolate lover myself, I do enjoy a piece of healthy chocolate every now and then. Healthy chocolate you say? Yes you heard that right. One of the biggest problems with chocolate is the heavy processing it goes through and the added sugar.

The raw Cacao Bean is one of nature's most fantastic superfoods due to its mineral content and wide array of unique and varied properties. Since many of the special properties of cacao are destroyed or lost by cooking, refining, and processing, we feel that planet Earth's favorite food is still unknown to most of us. Now we get to reconnect with the power of real chocolate: raw Cacao Beans.

With Cacao Beans there is fantastic hope for chocoholics everywhere! You can turn cravings for cooked, processed, chocolate into super-nutrition with raw chocolate (Cacao Beans).

Cacao Beans are extraordinarily nutritious!

Agave Syrup

Agave syrup is neither healthy nor natural (as many people believe it to be). Dr. Ingrid Kohlstadt, an associate faculty member at Johns Hopkins School of Public Health, stated "Agave is almost all fructose, a highly processed sugar with great marketing." There may be some vendors out there who are selling the real deal, but many agave sellers are actually selling a highly processed sugar that is even worse for you than high fructose corn syrup.

Action Steps

- Read labels! The sugar content of any food is listed right under the carbohydrate listing. Also pay attention to where the sugar is listed in the ingredients. (The order indicates relative quantity.)

- Avoid all foods that contain artificial sweeteners, sugar, or sugar derivatives.

- Avoid all sweetened beverages, including fruit juices that are not freshly juiced.

- For all your baking and sweetening needs, stevia and raw organic cacao are the best choices.

14: Alcohol

Because alcohol is extremely detrimental to health as well as weight-loss efforts, you must understand just how bad it is.

You may have heard that certain types of alcohol are good for your heart and reduce cholesterol levels. Unfortunately, because of its high calorie content and toxic effects on the liver, alcohol does not support weight-loss efforts. I also argue that wine consumption could negatively affect heart function more than help it.

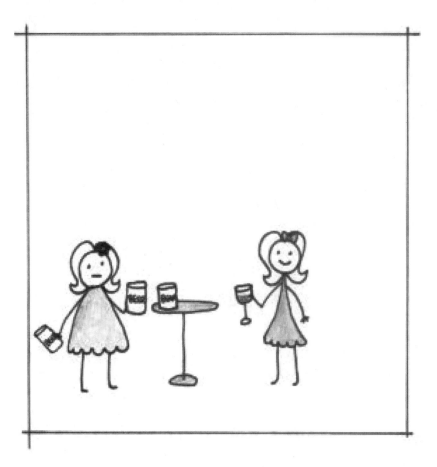

A standard mixed alcoholic drink contains 100–250 calories, but that's only part of the problem. Most people eat more when they drink. So although you may rationalize your drink choice by thinking that you will eat less at dinner, it rarely works that way. Alcohol often makes you crave the foods you should avoid: more carbohydrates and sugar. It also may cause you to eat unhealthy foods the day after, if you feel groggy and dehydrated. Why drink something that will make it difficult for you to make healthy choices?

Alcohol is considered a carbohydrate, but your body processes it differently from other carbohydrates. Made from fermented wheat, barley, grapes, or some other carbohydrate (e.g., potatoes), alcohol contains 7 calories per gram, compared with 4 calories per gram in most carbohydrates. The human body treats alcohol as a toxin, and as a result, the liver processes alcohol calories before all others in an attempt to clean the toxins from the bloodstream. As other calories wait on line, so to speak, the body senses a rise in calories and stores many of them away in fat cells, which is exactly what you don't want when you're trying to lose weight.

In short, alcohol is the absolute worst beverage you can drink when you are trying to control the amount and types of carbohydrates in your diet. For all the reasons stated here and more, keep alcohol consumption to an absolute minimum while on a weight-loss program (Kirsch 2005). After you have improved your eating habits, your body will become unable to handle as much alcohol as it did before, and you'll likely feel better overall without it. As a result, most people find that they feel best drinking no more than one glass of wine with dinner, on occasion.

I am sure you are familiar with the old saying, "It's not what you do between Christmas and New Year's, but what you do between New Year's and Christmas." An occasional indulgence every now and then won't hurt you. Just beware of the consequences. Once your body gets used to eating healthy regularly, you may experience discomfort when you indulge, such as stomach pain, bloating, or even a skin rash.

As for alcohol, there are healthier options. For instance, organic wines such as Frey are free of sulfites. Other suggestions are Skyy vodka, which is free of sulfites or unpasteurized sake. If you are still trying to lose weight, limit yourself to one or two drinks.

Action Steps

- While following this program to lose weight, drink no more than one glass per week, or, preferably, eliminate alcohol completely.

- If you drink alcohol, choose organic red wine. The rich flavor encourages you to drink slowly. Red wine also contains fewer calories and carbohydrates than other types of alcohol.

- A second-choice alcohol option is vodka on the rocks; fruit juice only adds empty sugar calories. The best brand is Chopin, which is made from potatoes, not wheat.

- After you reach your ideal weight, you can be a little more lenient, but minimize alcohol consumption to maintain a healthy weight.

15: Supplements

The diet industry has falsely led many people to believe that in order to lose weight successfully, they have to take a load of pills, eat special "diet foods" and/or drink certain "diet shakes." None of this is true, and you will see throughout this program that I make very few recommendations for supplements, and they are not required to make this program successful.

I would like to first emphasize that nothing can replace the nutritional value of real wholesome food. There may be some places in your eating plan where a supplement can prove helpful, but you always want to remember "real food is the best food."

With that being said, I do believe there are a few supplements that are worth consideration by most people and that I take myself each day. Below I have given you the supplements that I have thoroughly researched and tested and feel good about recommending to my family, friends, readers and clients.

Fish Oil

My personal recommendation for fish oil is BioTrust OmegaKrill 5X (http://go.beyonddiet.com/biotrustomegakrill). BioTrust is a reputable company, and I personally worked with the owners to create the highest-quality krill oil product. They are just as passionate about their work as I am about mine, and I know they stand behind the quality of their products.

This is one of the highest quality fish oil/krill oil combination Omega-3 supplements on the market today. It is the one my husband and I take every single day. It uses a special advanced absorption technology that ensures your body is absorbing and effectively using the oils contained in the product. It also does NOT give you those icky "fishy burps" that many other Omega-3 supplements give. Also, OmegaKrill 5X is free of any mercury or toxic chemicals (this is not something I can say about most brands on the market today).

Krill oil has also been found to accelerate the fat burning process in our bodies. More good news for those on a weight loss plan.

Protein Supplements

Protein Bars
I do not use or recommend protein bars in my nutrition practice. Most bars contain soy protein which is extremely harmful to the body and can cause weight gain in many people. Many bars also contain preservatives to increase their shelf life. With wonderful, healthy "on the go" choices like raw nuts and fresh fruits, there is no need to depend on artificial food like protein bars for snacks.

Protein Powders
Many people like to use protein powders as a quick and easy form of protein. I urge you to always go for food sources of protein first (eggs, poultry, meats, fish), but when you are in the mood for a smoothie or need a quick shake in between meals, there is only 1 protein powder I feel good recommending.

The only protein powder I recommend is BioTrust Protein Powder (http://go.beyonddiet.com/biotrustproteinpowder). BioTrust has formulated, what I feel, is one of the best protein powders on the market. Not only is it the best tasting protein powder I've ever had, it is made from 100% natural ingredients, with no artificial additives or toxic ingredients contained in most protein powders. This protein powder is sourced from grass fed cows that were raised naturally (not many companies can say that about their protein powders) and is sweetened with Stevia. Finally, BioTrust Protein Powder contains ProHydrolase, a digestive enzyme that specifically breaks down whey protein in the body, preventing any gas or bloating while simultaneously DOUBLING your body's ability to absorb and make best use of this protein.

Greens Powder
For those who have a difficult time getting in enough servings of fruits and vegetables each day, a greens food powder is a good choice. My personal favorite is Athletic Greens (http://go.beyonddiet.com/athleticgreens) and I drink one serving each and every day. It contains 76, all natural ingredients, most of which are organic. Athletic Greens is also packed with digestive enzymes, prebiotics and probiotics that all work together to

improve digestions and gastrointestinal function. It contains absolutely no synthetic chemicals, artificial colors, flavors, preservatives or sweeteners of any kind, no GMO's, herbicides, or pesticides, no wheat, dairy, gluten, corn, lactose, sucrose, dextrose, egg, yeast, or peanuts and no animal products.

Fat Burning Pills

Fat burning pills are downright dangerous and can cause severe side effects and even death, in extreme cases. Fat burning pills unnaturally elevate your heart rate and blood pressure, and can become addictive very quickly. Many people who have used fat burning pills to lose weight, almost always gain it back, sometimes more than they initially lost. Stay away from fat burning pills at all costs.

Action Steps

- Eat healthy foods that will supply you with the vitamins and nutrients you need.

- One of the best ways to improve your health with a supplement is increasing your intake of omega-3 fatty acids. BioTrust is an excellent source for this. You can purchase BioTrust OmegaKrill 5X online.

- Avoid any and all fat burning pills!

16: Vegetarians

I do believe that most people can greatly benefit from eating natural sources of animal proteins like grass fed beef, free range poultry and wild fish. Many fears vegetarians have around eating meats are the toxic and dangerous antibiotics and hormones that are added to conventional animal products. That is why I strongly recommend finding meat sources that are natural, free range, with no added antibiotics and hormones.

As much as I would love to urge everyone to include some animal products into their eating plan, being vegetarian is a personal choice and one that I do respect.

Below I have included some alternative options for vegetarians when following the program. I have seen many vegetarian readers experience great success with these modifications: losing weight, experiencing increased energy, and reversing health problems.

Depending on what type of vegetarian you are, your protein choices can include:

- eggs

- wild fish

- cottage cheese

- all varieties of raw nuts

- all varieties of raw nut butters

- all legumes*

*Vegetarians can take all of the beans and legumes listed in the "Carb Choices Chart" and make them part of their "Protein Choices Chart." This will not affect the success of the program in any way. For example, instead of having 1/2 cup of garbanzo beans be a Carb choice, it will now count as a Protein choice for that meal.

Below are some meal examples that show you how you can include a protein option (as listed above) into each and every meal.

Vegetarian breakfasts may include:

- Oatmeal with almond butter and fresh fruit

- Cottage Cheese over fruit salad with walnuts sprinkled on top

- Homemade Hummus on sprouted whole grain toast

Vegetarian snacks may include

- Baby carrots and sliced red peppers dipped in almond, peanut or walnut butter

- Raw Brazil nuts and sliced apple

- Homemade Hummus with sliced cucumbers

Vegetarian lunches and dinners may include:

- Kidney Bean and Mushroom Veggie Burger or Garbanzo Bean Burger over sauteed greens with slices of tomato on top with brown rice

- Veggie Vegetarian Chili over shredded lettuce and a sprouted grain tortilla

- Lentil and Vegetable Soup

17: Conditions and Illnesses

I am allergic to many foods. Will this program still work for me?

As with any meal plan, please stay away from those foods listed you are allergic to. Often people with allergies to wheat, gluten, and dairy do quite well on The DSP because these foods are not emphasized on this plan. On the contrary, I suggest most people (even those without allergies) eliminate these foods from their meal plans.

If you are allergic to peanuts and/or tree nuts, you can still have much success on this program as there are many other healthy protein choices available.

I have Celiac disease. Will this program work for me?

I think you will actually find that the meal plans will be particularly helpful for those with Celiac disease. I actually recommend that most people stay away from most grains (especially those containing gluten) and they will lose weight and feel so much better without them. If you must eliminate gluten containing foods from your daily meal plan, you will be able to do that easily on this program.

My doctor has me on a specific diet. How can I modify my Beyond Diet meals accordingly

Of course, you must always adhere to your doctor's prescriptions and suggestions. If your doctor has you on a specific diet eliminating certain foods, you should eliminate those foods from your food choices list. For example, there are some medications that require some people to stay away from certain leafy greens or citrus fruits like grapefruit and oranges. If you happen to be one of those people, eliminate those foods from your suggested meal plans and replace them with a different vegetable and/or different fruit.

Most doctors would agree that the natural foods and the meal plans suggested in the Program are a healthy way for anyone to eat, especially those who need to reduce their weight for medical reasons. These plans have helped many people reduce their cholesterol, control their diabetes and reduce inflammation from conditions like arthritis and fibromyalgia.

I suggest you create your meal plans and bring them to your doctor. Ask him or her if the foods included on your plan are a healthy option for you.

Can this program help with Arthritis?

Yes, you will receive a great benefit from the program as it recommends inflammation-lowering foods. Start off by eliminating dairy and wheat from your diet and you will already start to feel better.

Can I follow this plan if I have Type I or II Diabetes?

This program is perfect for Diabetics! Not only will assist in stabilizing your blood sugar, it will help you lose weight at the same time. As far as controlling diabetes, the best thing to do would be to determine your Metabolism Type and then follow the No-Grains Meal Plans for that type. This has proved successful with many of my clients. Making your primary source of carbohydrates vegetables and fruits helps to keep blood sugar much more controlled.

18: Incorporating BD Into Your Life

Do I have to read the entire manual before I begin?

No, you do not need to read the entire manual start to finish before getting started on your new weight loss plan. I have made sure to provide you with all of the tools and necessary information to create the best weight loss plan for you. This is why there is what my seem to be a lot of reading material. But don't worry. There is a quick and easy way to get started on your goals without having to read the entire manual all at once.

Begin by reading through the Quick Start Guide. I have made each topic easy to read and simple to understand in order to help you get started as quickly as possible. The next step is to follow the 14 Days of Supercharged Meal Plans. These meal plans are on the simple side, but they will be very effective at launching your progress to your new body. Don't worry, we will get into fancier and more complex meals and recipes soon, but this will give you the jumpstart you are looking for.

Once you have read the Quick Start and completed the 14 Days of Supercharged Meal Plans, it's time to have you understand the underlying principles of Beyond Diet so you can enjoy making eating this way part of your own lifestyle. Read the Main Manual which will walk you through all the tools and information you need to know to keep losing fat and maintain the body you've been looking for.

Can I really stick to this plan even with my busy lifestyle?

Absolutely! This program will teach you how a healthy eating plan is possible with any lifestyle, even those who are always on the go. You can stick to any plan with the right commitment and preparation. Once you know which foods are best for you and your goals, you can then easily find these foods in supermarkets and restaurants that are most convenient to you. For example, if you are on the go and have not prepared your food ahead of time, you can stop at any supermarket and get raw nuts, fresh fruits or a salad and prepared meat, poultry or fish from the salad bar. The trick is to know which foods you are looking for so you can make good choices even when you are on the go.

What if I am not hungry for every one of my meals?

You can always tailor the program to best suit your needs. As long as you are eating the recommended foods and staying away from processed and artificial foods, you can plan your meals according to what feels best to you. If eating a few less meals a day works better for you, you can most definitely do that. Just make sure not to be hungry or starve your body throughout the day.

If you are not hungry for your mid morning or mid afternoon snack, pay attention to your body and never force feed it. You may find that just 5-6 almonds between meals is enough to get you to lunch or dinner without feeling uncomfortably full. Most importantly do not skip your snacks in an effort to lose more weight. If your body is hungry, it is telling you it needs a bit more food. Not to mention, your metabolism will continue to work all day long as you feed it healthy foods throughout the day.

What should I do if I'm hungry during the day or at night?

If you experience hunger while following Beyond Diet, pay close attention to your body's cues. If you are hungry, it means you may have not eaten a sufficient amount of food or you ate enough food but in the wrong combination. Snack on healthy food choices like raw almonds, sliced apples, or slices of fresh turkey. Turn to foods with a higher protein content as they are the most filling and will better combat "in between meals" hunger.

Can my children and the rest of my family also follow these meal plans?

Yes, and I highly recommend you feed your children and the rest of your family the foods and meal plans taught in Beyond Diet. The principles taught in Beyond Diet are the foundation to any healthy eating plan. It is by no means a crash diet or extreme meal plan that is unsafe for anyone. I do recommend catering the portions to each individual. You may find that your children may need more or less food than you to feel energetic and satiated.

What if I can't find certain foods in my geographic location?

I understand that certain cities and countries may all have different foods available. You can make adjustments to your meal plans based on the foods you have available to you. You may also want to search the internet to see if there are some foods and products you can order online and have mailed directly to your home. Please be sure to take a look at The Shopping Guide and my recommended products online at http://go.beyonddiet.com/shopping

Remember, you do not need to make this program "all or nothing." By that I mean, you will still see great weight loss results by implementing even just a few of the recommended action steps. Modify your meal plans to work best with the foods you have available and remember to make eating wholesome natural foods your first priority.

How much does sleep affect my weight loss?

If your body is sleep deprived, you may have difficulty losing weight or, worse, gain weight. Many people, including myself, tend to crave "sugar" foods when they are tired and deprived of sleep to get them through the day. This often leads to a roller coaster ride of sugar highs and lows, on top of an already exhausted body.

Our hormones are also affected by our sleep patterns. Lack of sleep increases levels of the hormone grehlin, which **increases appetite,** while decreasing levels of the hormone leptin, which **makes people feel full**.

These hormone fluctuations combined with feelings of exhaustion make sticking to a healthy eating plan much more challenging.

Can stress be causing me to not lose weight or gain weight?

Yes. Stress is many times the reason most people cannot shed their unwanted pounds [kilos]. The more obvious reason is many people turn to food for comfort when they are stressed. This does nothing, but usually make the situation worse, as they are now still stressed and not feeling good about themselves.

Hormonally, stress has been found to increase levels of cortisol in the body for extended periods of time. Cortisol's job is to replenish the body after the stress has passed, often hanging around much longer than we would like. It significantly increases appetite to ensure that our bodies are well nourished after a stressful event. Unfortunately, in today's society, it is usually not just one stressful event, but a continuous stressful life. This state often leads to consistent high levels of cortisol in the blood stream and constant feelings of hunger and cravings.

Can I use a microwave oven on this program?

I highly recommend people stay away from microwave ovens. Putting your foods through these dangerous microwave waves completely damages the molecular structure of the food you are heating up, making it unrecognizable to the body. Completely eliminating or greatly reducing the amount you use your microwave oven will have a significant positive impact on your health and you ability to lose weight.

What affect does chewing gum have on my metabolism?

The biggest problem with chewing gum is that most gums contains aspartame and many unnatural chemicals. Also, people who chew lots of gum during the day usually complain of gas and bloating. I would keep gum chewing to a minimum of 1-2 pieces per week or none at all.

Do I need to stick with the specific brands of food you mention?

No, you don't need to stick to the specific brands for Beyond Diet to still be effective. As long as you have access to fresh fruits, vegetables, natural proteins, and raw nuts, you can have much success on The Program.

Should I do a detox before starting this program?

No. A detox is not necessary to begin starting The Beyond Diet Program. You will find that by following the principles outlined in the manual, you will naturally be de-toxifying your body from harmful substances that are in processed foods, refined grains, sugar, and artificial sweeteners.

Will your program get rid of my cellulite?

Cellulite is your body's way of storing toxins in your fat cells. The only way to rid your body of this cellulite is to first rid your body of these toxins. Once your body sees a decreased amount of toxins in your body, it will eliminate this unwanted fat. The best recipe for ridding your body of cellulite is to eat wholesome, natural foods, eliminate processed foods, and follow a consistent exercise routine that include strength training and cardiovascular exercise.

I am trying to put on muscle mass. Will these meal plans help me with that?

Yes. Beyond Diet does include a sufficient amount of protein for men and women to put on muscle mass. My only suggestion would be to increase your protein serving by 1-2 servings and increase your complex carb serving in your post workout meal. For example, having a bit more chicken and an extra serving of sweet potato or brown rice would be great after a strength training workout.

You may also want to adjust your calorie calculations. Instead of subtracting 20% from your baseline calories, you may want to add 20%. For example, a very active male who wishes to gain weight, primarily in the form of muscle, would multiply his current weight by 15, multiply this number by 20%, and then add that total to the initial calorie calculation.

How can I maintain muscle while losing weight?

In order to maintain your current muscle mass while still burning unwanted fat, you may want to modify the calorie calculation a bit:

Instead of subtracting 20% from your baseline calories, you will add 20%. For example, a very active male who wishes to gain weight, primarily in the form of muscle, would multiply his current weight by 15, multiply this number by 20%, and then add that total to the initial calorie calculation.

You may also want to choose the "no grain" meal plans as they result in faster fat loss while still maintaining a sufficient amount of protein for muscle retention.

19: Guides & Charts

Cooking with Fats

The following guide to commonly used culinary fats will help you choose the proper fats for each type of cooking according to their smoke points (Chek 2004, 73). Always use unrefined organic oils and raw organic butter!

No-heat fats should never be used for cooking:
- borage oil
- fish oil or cod liver oil
- flax seed oil
- hemp seed oil

Low-heat fats should be heated to no more than 212°F:
- pumpkin oil
- safflower oil
- sunflower oil

Medium-heat fats should be heated to no more than 325°F (light sautéing):
- hazelnut oil
- olive oil
- pistachio oil
- sesame oil

High-heat fats should be heated to no more than 375°F (frying or browning):
- butter (for cooking at medium-high heat only; do not allow to turn brown)
- coconut oil
- ghee or clarified butter

Glycemic Index Chart

	INDEX	SUGAR	DAIRY	FRUIT	GRAIN	VEGETABLES
HIGH	>100	maltose beer alcohol		Date		Parsnip
	90–99	glucose sports drinks			instant rice puffed rice	
	80–89	jelly beans			Rice Chex, white rice pretzels, Rice Krispies Cornflakes, Rice Cakes	potato (white, baked) potato (white, instant mashed)
	70–79	Life Savers jams, jellies		watermelon	wheat cereal graham crackers Cheerios, bagels whole wheat bread white bread, millet	pumpkin rutabaga
MEDIUM	60–69	Honey		melon (all types) pineapple, raisin banana (ripe) apricot, mango	cornmeal rye crisp bread shredded wheat brown rice, brown rice pasta	Beet
	50–59			kiwifruit	corn popcorn oatmeal buckwheat	potato (sweet) yam carrot green peas
LOW	40–49	Lactose		grape orange	wheat bran bulgur wheat whole wheat pasta	beans (pinto or baked)
	30–39		yogurt whole milk butter	apple, pear strawberry	rye	tomato soup beans (navy, lima, black, or garbanzo) peas (black-eyed or dried split)
	<30	Fructose		peach grapefruit plum cherry tomato	barley rice bran	beans (kidney or lentil) peas (dried) eggplant, summer squash cauliflower, peanut green vegetables[a]

Notes: On the GI scale, high-GI foods are rapid insulin inducers and should be avoided; low-GI foods are slow insulin inducers and your best choices for weight loss.

[a] Vegetables with a GI of ~15 are ideal carbohydrate servings: artichoke, asparagus, broccoli, celery, cucumber, green bean, lettuce, green bell pepper, spinach, and zucchini.

Source: Adapted from Wolcott and Fahey 2000, 272–274.

Allowable Servings Guide

Type	Mixed	Carb	Protein
Meal	**1,400 calories/day**		
Breakfast	2 Protein 2 Carb	1 Protein 2 Carb	3 Protein 1 Carb
Snack	2 Protein 2 Carb	1 Protein 2 Carb	2 Protein 1 Carb
Lunch	3 Protein 1 Carb 1 Fat	3 Protein 2 Carb 1 Fat	3 Protein 1 Carb 2 Fat
Snack	2 Protein 1 Carb	2 Protein 2 Carb	2 Protein 1 Carb
Dinner	3 Protein 2 Carb 2 Fat	3 Protein 2 Carb 1 Fat	4 Protein 1 Carb 2 Fat
	1,600 calories/day		
Breakfast	2 Protein 2 Carb	1 Protein 2 Carb	3 Protein 1 Carb
Snack	2 Protein 2 Carb	1 Protein 2 Carb	2 Protein 1 Carb
Lunch	4 Protein 1 Carb 1 Fat	4 Protein 2 Carb 1 Fat	4 Protein 1 Carb 2 Fat
Snack	2 Protein 1 Carb	2 Protein 2 Carb	2 Protein 1 Carb
Dinner	4 Protein 2 Carb 2 Fat	4 Protein 2 Carb 1 Fat	5 Protein 1 Carb 2 Fat

Note: **Refer to the Food Choice charts to choose the appropriate foods in each category for your metabolism type.**

Allowable Servings Guide (cont.)

Type	Mixed	Carb	Protein
Meal	**1,800 calories/day**		
Breakfast	2 Protein 2 Carb	1 Protein 2 Carb	3 Protein 1 Carb
Snack	2 Protein 2 Carb	2 Protein 2 Carb	3 Protein 1 Carb
Lunch	4 Protein 2 Carb 1 Fat	4 Protein 2 Carb 1 Fat	4 Protein 1 Carb 2 Fat
Snack	2 Protein 1 Carb	2 Protein 3 Carb	2 Protein 1 Carb
Dinner	5 Protein 2 Carb 2 Fat	4 Protein 2 Carb 1 Fat	5 Protein 1 Carb 2 Fat
	2,000 calories/day		
Breakfast	3 Protein 2 Carb	2 Protein 3 Carb	3 Protein 1 Carb
Snack	2 Protein 2 Carb	2 Protein 2 Carb	3 Protein 1 Carb
Lunch	4 Protein 2 Carb 1 Fat	4 Protein 2 Carb 1 Fat	5 Protein 1 Carb 2 Fat
Snack	2 Protein 1 Carb	2 Protein 3 Carb	3 Protein 1 Carb
Dinner	5 Protein 2 Carb 2 Fat	4 Protein 2 Carb 1 Fat	5 Protein 1 Carb 2 Fat

Note: **Refer to the Food Choice charts to choose the appropriate foods in each category for your metabolism type.**

Allowable Servings Guide (cont.)

Type	Mixed	Carb	Protein
Meal	**2,200 calories/day**		
Breakfast	3 Protein 2 Carb	2 Protein 3 Carb	4 Protein 1 Carb
Snack	3 Protein 2 Carb	2 Protein 3 Carb	3 Protein 1 Carb
Lunch	4 Protein 2 Carb 1 Fat	4 Protein 3 Carb 1 Fat	5 Protein 1 Carb 2 Fat
Snack	2 Protein 2 Carb	2 Protein 3 Carb	4 Protein 1 Carb
Dinner	5 Protein 2 Carb 2 Fat	4 Protein 2 Carb 1 Fat	5 Protein 1 Carb 2 Fat
	2,400 calories/day		
Breakfast	3 Protein 2 Carb	2 Protein 3 Carb	4 Protein 2 Carb
Snack	3 Protein 2 Carb	2 Protein 3 Carb	3 Protein 1 Carb
Lunch	4 Protein 3 Carb 2 Fat	4 Protein 3 Carb 2 Fat	5 Protein 1 Carb 2 Fat
Snack	3 Protein 2 Carb	2 Protein 3 Carb	4 Protein 1 Carb
Dinner	5 Protein 2 Carb 2 Fat	4 Protein 3 Carb 1 Fat	6 Protein 1 Carb 2 Fat

Note: **Refer to the Food Choice charts to choose the appropriate foods in each category for your metabolism type.**

Food Choices

For all charts in this section, the "best bet" food items are shaded in gray.

Carb Types: Protein Choices

Serving	Meats	Serving	Seafood	Serving	Nuts[a] and Seeds
1 slice	bacon (pork)	1 oz (28g)	cod	½ oz (14g)	almonds
1 slice	bacon (beef)	1 oz (28g)	crabmeat	½ oz (14g)	Brazil nuts
1 oz (28g)	beef	1 oz (28g)	crayfish	½ oz (14g)	cashews
1 oz (28g)	buffalo	1 oz (28g)	flounder	½ oz (14g)	chestnuts
1 oz (28g)	lamb	1 oz (28g)	grouper	½ oz (14g)	filberts
1 oz (28g)	liver (beef or chicken)	1 oz (28g)	halibut	½ oz (14g)	hickory nuts
1 oz (28g)	pork (lean)	1 oz (28g)	herring	½ oz (14g)	macadamia nuts
1 oz (28g)	rabbit	1 oz (28g)	lobster meat	½ oz (14g)	peanuts[b]
1 oz (28g)	venison	1 oz (28g)	mackerel	½ oz (14g)	pecans
	Poultry	1 oz (28g)	mahimahi	½ oz (14g)	pine nuts
1 slice	bacon (turkey)	1 oz (28g)	mussels	½ oz (14g)	pistachios
1 oz (28g)	chicken (dark)	1 oz (28g)	octopus	½ oz (14g)	pumpkin seeds
1 oz (28g)	chicken (white)	1 oz (28g)	perch (freshwater)	½ oz (14g)	sunflower seeds
1 oz (28g)	duck	1 oz (28g)	rockfish	1 tbsp (15 mL)	nut butter[c]
1 oz (28g)	goose	1 oz (28g)	roughy		
1 oz (28g)	Cornish hen	1 oz (28g)	salmon		
1 oz (28g)	pheasant	1 oz (28g)	sardines		
1 oz (28g)	quail	1 oz (28g)	scallops		
1 oz (28g)	sausage (chicken)	1 oz (28g)	shark		
1 oz (28g)	turkey (dark)	1 oz (28g)	shrimp		
1 oz (28g)	turkey (white)	1 oz (28g)	snapper		
	Seafood	1 oz (28g)	squid		
1 oz (28g)	abalone	1 oz (28g)	swordfish		
1 oz (28g)	anchovy	1 oz (28g)	trout		
1 oz (28g)	bass (freshwater)	1 oz (28g)	tuna (white)		
1 oz (28g)	bass (sea)	1 oz (28g)	whitefish		
1 oz (28g)	catfish		**Dairy and Eggs**		
1 oz (28g)	caviar	1	egg		
1 oz (28g)	clams	¼ cup (60g)	cottage cheese (raw)		
		2 oz (56g)	greek yogurt		

[a] All nuts and seeds must be raw.
[b] Peanuts are legumes but are listed with tree nuts here for ease of presentation.
[c] Varieties of nut butter include almond, cashew, macadamia nut, and walnut.

Carb Types: Carbohydrate Choices

Serving	Legumes*	Serving	Low-Starch Veg*	Serving	Low-Starch Veg*
½ cup (75g)	adzuki beans	1	artichoke	½ cup (75g)	turnip
½ cup (75g)	black beans	1 cup (150g)	asparagus	1 cup (150g)	zucchini
½ cup (75g)	black-eyed beans	½ cup (75g)	bamboo shoots		
½ cup (75g)	fava beans	1 cup (150g)	bok choy		
½ cup (75g)	garbanzo beans	1 cup (150g)	broccoli		
½ cup (75g)	great Northern beans	1 cup (150g)	brussels sprouts		
½ cup (75g)	green beans	1 cup (150g)	cabbage		
½ cup (75g)	green peas	1 cup (150g)	cauliflower		
½ cup (75g)	lentils	1 cup (150g)	celery		
½ cup (75g)	lima beans	1 cup (150g)	cucumber		
½ cup (75g)	mung beans	1 cup (150g)	daikon[a]		
½ cup (75g)	navy beans	1 cup (150g)	eggplant		
½ cup (75g)	pink beans	1 cup (150g)	fennel		
½ cup (75g)	pinto beans	free	garlic		
½ cup (75g)	red beans	free	gingerroot		
½ cup (75g)	white beans	1 cup (150g)	jicama		
	High-Starch Veg*	1 cup (150g)	kale		
1 cup (150g)	beets	free	lettuce[d]		
1 cup (150g)	carrots	1 cup (150g)	mushrooms		
½ cup (75g)	Jerusalem artichoke	1 cup (150g)	okra		
½ cup (75g)	parsnips	5	olives		
½ cup (75g)	potato (white)	1	onion (medium)		
½ cup (75g)	potato (sweet)	1 cup (150g)	pepper (bell)		
¼ cup (60g)	water chestnuts	free	pepper (hot)		
	Dairy	½ cup (75g)	pumpkin		
½ cup (75g)	milk (raw)	½ cup (75g)	radishes		
6 oz (168g)	plain yogurt	½ cup (75g)	rutabaga[e]		
		1 cup (150g)	salad greens[d]		
		1 cup (150g)	spinach		
		½ cup (75g)	squash (winter)[f]		

Notes: *Serving sizes of grains and legumes are measured cooked; those of fruits and vegetables are measured raw.

**SWG = sprouted whole grain (e.g., Ezekiel 4:9 products).

Free = Use as needed for seasoning.

[a] Japanese radish.
[b] Similar to an orange but small like a grape.
[c] Cross between a blackberry and raspberry.
[d] Any but iceberg.
[e] Similar to a turnip.
[f] Orange-fleshed squashes (e.g., acorn, butternut, and kabocha).
[g] Similar to a cantaloupe.

Carb Types: Carbohydrate Choices

Serving	Bread	Serving	Fruits (cont.)	Serving	Fruits (cont.)
1 slice	SWG** bread	1 cup (150g)	casaba melon[g]	2 cups (300g)	rhubarb
½	SWG** roll	17	cherries	1 cup (150g)	strawberries
1	SWG** English muffin	1 cup (150g)	cranberries	2	tangerines (small)
1	SWG** wrap (small)	1 cup (150g)	currants	1	tomato (large)
1 slice	rice bread	1	date	1 cup (150g)	watermelon
1 slice	spelt bread	¾ cup (111g)	elderberries		
10	rice crackers	2	figs (large)		
2	rye crackers	1 cup (150g)	gooseberries		
	Grains*	1	grapefruit (small)		
½ cup (75g)	brown or wild rice	17-20	grapes		
½ cup (75g)	amaranth	1 cup (150g)	guava		
½ cup (75g)	barley	1 cup (150g)	honeydew melon		
½ cup (75g)	buckwheat	2	kiwifruit (medium)		
½ cup (75g)	corn	6	kumquat[b]		
½ cup (75g)	kamut	free	lemons		
½ cup (75g)	millet	free	limes		
1 cup (150g)	oatmeal	1 cup (150g)	loganberries[c]		
½ cup (75g)	quinoa	½	mango		
½ cup (75g)	rye	2	nectarines (small)		
½ cup (75g)	spelt	1	orange (large)		
½ cup (75g)	SWG** cereal	½	papaya (large)		
½ cup (75g)	raw granola	1	peach (medium)		
	Fruits*	1	pear (medium)		
1	apple (medium)	2	persimmons		
4	apricots (small)	1 cup (150g)	pineapple		
½	banana (medium)	2	plums (small)		
1 cup (150g)	blackberries	1	pomegranate (small)		
1 cup (150g)	blueberries	4	prunes (small)		
1 cup (150g)	boysenberries	¼ cup (60g)	Raisins		
1 cup (150g)	cantaloupe	1 cup (150g)	raspberries		

Notes: *Serving sizes of grains and legumes are measured cooked; those of fruits and vegetables are measured raw.

**SWG = sprouted whole grain (e.g., Ezekiel 4:9 products).

Free = Use as needed for seasoning.

[a] Japanese radish.

[b] Similar to an orange but small like a grape.

[c] Cross between a blackberry and raspberry.

[d] Any but iceberg.

[e] Similar to a turnip.

[f] Orange-fleshed squashes (e.g., acorn, butternut, and kabocha).

[g] Similar to a cantaloupe.

Protein Types: Protein Choices

Serving	Meats	Serving	Seafood	Serving	Nuts[a] and Seeds
1 slice	bacon (pork)	1 oz (28g)	cod	½ oz (14g)	almonds
1 slice	bacon (beef)	1 oz (28g)	crabmeat	½ oz (14g)	Brazil nuts
1 oz (28g)	beef	1 oz (28g)	crayfish	½ oz (14g)	cashews
1 oz (28g)	buffalo	1 oz (28g)	flounder	½ oz (14g)	chestnuts
1 oz (28g)	lamb	1 oz (28g)	grouper	½ oz (14g)	filberts
1 oz (28g)	liver (beef or chicken)	1 oz (28g)	halibut	½ oz (14g)	hickory nuts
1 oz (28g)	pork (lean)	1 oz (28g)	herring	½ oz (14g)	macadamia nuts
1 oz (28g)	rabbit	1 oz (28g)	lobster meat	½ oz (14g)	peanuts[b]
1 oz (28g)	venison	1 oz (28g)	mackerel	½ oz (14g)	pecans
	Poultry	1 oz (28g)	mahimahi	½ oz (14g)	pine nuts
1 slice	bacon (turkey)	1 oz (28g)	mussels	½ oz (14g)	pistachios
1 oz (28g)	chicken (dark)	1 oz (28g)	octopus	½ oz (14g)	pumpkin seeds
1 oz (28g)	chicken (white)	1 oz (28g)	perch (ocean)	½ oz (14g)	sunflower seeds
1 oz (28g)	duck	1 oz (28g)	rockfish	1 tbsp (15 mL)	nut butter[c]
1 oz (28g)	goose	1 oz (28g)	roughy		
1 oz (28g)	Cornish hen	1 oz (28g)	salmon		
1 oz (28g)	pheasant	1 oz (28g)	sardines		
1 oz (28g)	quail	1 oz (28g)	scallops		
1 oz (28g)	sausage (chicken)	1 oz (28g)	shark		
1 oz (28g)	turkey (dark)	1 oz (28g)	shrimp		
1 oz (28g)	turkey (white)	1 oz (28g)	snapper		
	Seafood	1 oz (28g)	squid		
1 oz (28g)	abalone	1 oz (28g)	swordfish		
1 oz (28g)	anchovy	1 oz (28g)	trout		
1 oz (28g)	bass (freshwater)	1 oz (28g)	tuna (dark)		
1 oz (28g)	bass (sea)	1 oz (28g)	whitefish		
1 oz (28g)	catfish		**Dairy and Eggs**		
1 oz (28g)	caviar	1	egg		
1 oz (28g)	clams	¼ cup (60g)	cottage cheese (raw)		
		2 oz (56g)	greek yogurt		

[a] All nuts and seeds must be raw.
[b] Peanuts are legumes but are listed with tree nuts here for ease of presentation.
[c] Varieties of nut butter include almond, cashew, macadamia nut, and walnut.

Protein Types: Carbohydrate Choices

Serving	Bread	Serving	Fruits (cont.)	Serving	Fruits (cont.)
1 slice	SWG** bread	1 cup (150g)	casaba melon[g]	2 cups (300g)	rhubarb
½	SWG** roll	17	cherries	1 cup (150g)	strawberries
1	SWG** English muffin	1 cup (150g)	cranberries	2	tangerines (small)
1	SWG** wrap (small)	1 cup (150g)	currants	1	tomato (large)
1 slice	rice bread	1	date	1 cup (150g)	watermelon
1 slice	spelt bread	¾ cup (111g)	elderberries		
10	rice crackers	2	figs (large)		
2	rye crackers	1 cup (150g)	gooseberries		
	Grains*	1	grapefruit (small)		
½ cup (75g)	brown or wild rice	17-20	grapes		
½ cup (75g)	amaranth	1 cup (150g)	guava		
½ cup (75g)	barley	1 cup (150g)	honeydew melon		
½ cup (75g)	buckwheat	2	kiwifruit (medium)		
½ cup (75g)	corn	6	kumquat[b]		
½ cup (75g)	kamut	free	lemons		
½ cup (75g)	millet	free	limes		
1 cup (150g)	oatmeal	1 cup (150g)	loganberries[c]		
½ cup (75g)	quinoa	½	mango		
½ cup (75g)	rye	2	nectarines (small)		
½ cup (75g)	spelt	1	orange (large)		
½ cup (75g)	SWG** cereal	½	papaya (large)		
½ cup (75g)	raw granola	1	peach (medium)		
	Fruits*	1	pear (medium)		
1	apple (medium)	2	persimmons		
4	apricots (small)	1 cup (150g)	pineapple		
½	banana (medium)	2	plums (small)		
1 cup (150g)	blackberries	1	pomegranate (small)		
1 cup (150g)	blueberries	4	prunes (small)		
1 cup (150g)	boysenberries	¼ cup (60g)	Raisins		
1 cup (150g)	cantaloupe	1 cup (150g)	raspberries		

Notes: *Serving sizes of grains and legumes are measured cooked; those of fruits and vegetables are measured raw.

**SWG = sprouted whole grain (e.g., Ezekiel 4:9 products).

Free = Use as needed for seasoning.

[a] Japanese radish.

[b] Similar to an orange but small like a grape.

[c] Cross between a blackberry and raspberry.

[d] Any but iceberg.

[e] Similar to a turnip.

[f] Orange-fleshed squashes (e.g., acorn, butternut, and kabocha).

[g] Similar to a cantaloupe.

Protein Types: Carbohydrate Choices

Serving	Legumes*	Serving	Low-Starch Veg*	Serving	Low-Starch Veg*
½ cup (75g)	adzuki beans	1	artichoke	½ cup (75g)	turnip
½ cup (75g)	black beans	1 cup (150g)	asparagus	1 cup (150g)	zucchini
½ cup (75g)	black-eyed beans	½ cup (75g)	bamboo shoots		
½ cup (75g)	fava beans	1 cup (150g)	bok choy		
½ cup (75g)	garbanzo beans	1 cup (150g)	broccoli		
½ cup (75g)	great Northern beans	1 cup (150g)	brussels sprouts		
½ cup (75g)	green beans	1 cup (150g)	cabbage		
½ cup (75g)	green peas	1 cup (150g)	cauliflower		
½ cup (75g)	lentils	1 cup (150g)	celery		
½ cup (75g)	lima beans	1 cup (150g)	cucumber		
½ cup (75g)	mung beans	1 cup (150g)	daikon[a]		
½ cup (75g)	navy beans	1 cup (150g)	eggplant		
½ cup (75g)	pink beans	1 cup (150g)	fennel		
½ cup (75g)	pinto beans	free	garlic		
½ cup (75g)	red beans	free	gingerroot		
½ cup (75g)	white beans	1 cup (150g)	jicama		
	High-Starch Veg*	1 cup (150g)	kale		
1 cup (150g)	beets	free	lettuce[d]		
1 cup (150g)	carrots	1 cup (150g)	mushrooms		
½ cup (75g)	Jerusalem artichoke	1 cup (150g)	okra		
½ cup (75g)	parsnips	5	olives		
½ cup (75g)	potato (white)	1	onion (medium)		
½ cup (75g)	potato (sweet)	1 cup (150g)	pepper (bell)		
¼ cup (60g)	water chestnuts	free	pepper (hot)		
	Dairy	½ cup (75g)	pumpkin		
½ cup (75g)	milk (raw)	½ cup (75g)	radishes		
6 oz (168g)	plain yogurt	½ cup (75g)	rutabaga[e]		
		1 cup (150g)	salad greens[d]		
		1 cup (150g)	spinach		
		½ cup (75g)	squash (winter)[f]		

Notes: *Serving sizes of grains and legumes are measured cooked; those of fruits and vegetables are measured raw.

**SWG = sprouted whole grain (e.g., Ezekiel 4:9 products).

Free = Use as needed for seasoning.

[a] Japanese radish.

[b] Similar to an orange but small like a grape.

[c] Cross between a blackberry and raspberry.

[d] Any but iceberg.

[e] Similar to a turnip.

[f] Orange-fleshed squashes (e.g., acorn, butternut, and kabocha).

[g] Similar to a cantaloupe.

Mixed Types: Protein Choices

Serving	Meats	Serving	Seafood	Serving	Nuts[a] and Seeds
1 slice	bacon (pork)	1 oz (28g)	cod	½ oz (14g)	almonds
1 slice	bacon (beef)	1 oz (28g)	crabmeat	½ oz (14g)	Brazil nuts
1 oz (28g)	beef	1 oz (28g)	crayfish	½ oz (14g)	cashews
1 oz (28g)	buffalo	1 oz (28g)	flounder	½ oz (14g)	chestnuts
1 oz (28g)	lamb	1 oz (28g)	grouper	½ oz (14g)	filberts
1 oz (28g)	liver (beef or chicken)	1 oz (28g)	halibut	½ oz (14g)	hickory nuts
1 oz (28g)	pork (lean)	1 oz (28g)	herring	½ oz (14g)	macadamia nuts
1 oz (28g)	rabbit	1 oz (28g)	lobster meat	½ oz (14g)	peanuts[b]
1 oz (28g)	venison	1 oz (28g)	mackerel	½ oz (14g)	pecans
	Poultry	1 oz (28g)	mahimahi	½ oz (14g)	pine nuts
1 slice	bacon (turkey)	1 oz (28g)	mussels	½ oz (14g)	pistachios
1 oz (28g)	chicken (dark)	1 oz (28g)	octopus	½ oz (14g)	pumpkin seeds
1 oz (28g)	chicken (white)	1 oz (28g)	perch (ocean)	½ oz (14g)	sunflower seeds
1 oz (28g)	duck	1 oz (28g)	rockfish	1 tbsp (15 mL)	nut butter[c]
1 oz (28g)	goose	1 oz (28g)	roughy		
1 oz (28g)	Cornish hen	1 oz (28g)	salmon		
1 oz (28g)	pheasant	1 oz (28g)	sardines		
1 oz (28g)	quail	1 oz (28g)	scallops		
1 oz (28g)	sausage (chicken)	1 oz (28g)	shark		
1 oz (28g)	turkey (dark)	1 oz (28g)	shrimp		
1 oz (28g)	turkey (white)	1 oz (28g)	snapper		
	Seafood	1 oz (28g)	squid		
1 oz (28g)	abalone	1 oz (28g)	swordfish		
1 oz (28g)	anchovy	1 oz (28g)	trout		
1 oz (28g)	bass (freshwater)	1 oz (28g)	tuna (dark)		
1 oz (28g)	bass (sea)	1 oz (28g)	whitefish		
1 oz (28g)	catfish		**Dairy and Eggs**		
1 oz (28g)	caviar	1	egg		
1 oz (28g)	clams	¼ cup (60g)	cottage cheese (raw)		
		2 oz (56g)	greek yogurt		

[a] All nuts and seeds must be raw.
[b] Peanuts are legumes but are listed with tree nuts here for ease of presentation.
[c] Varieties of nut butter include almond, cashew, macadamia nut, and walnut.

Mixed Types: Carbohydrate Choices

Serving	Bread	Serving	Fruits (cont.)	Serving	Fruits (cont.)
1 slice	SWG** bread	1 cup (150g)	casaba melon[g]	2 cups (300g)	rhubarb
½	SWG** roll	17	cherries	1 cup (150g)	strawberries
1	SWG** English muffin	1 cup (150g)	cranberries	2	tangerines (small)
1	SWG** wrap (small)	1 cup (150g)	currants	1	tomato (large)
1 slice	rice bread	1	date	1 cup (150g)	watermelon
1 slice	spelt bread	¾ cup (111g)	elderberries		
10	rice crackers	2	figs (large)		
2	rye crackers	1 cup (150g)	gooseberries		
	Grains*	1	grapefruit (small)		
½ cup (75g)	brown or wild rice	17-20	grapes		
½ cup (75g)	amaranth	1 cup (150g)	guava		
½ cup (75g)	barley	1 cup (150g)	honeydew melon		
½ cup (75g)	buckwheat	2	kiwifruit (medium)		
½ cup (75g)	corn	6	kumquat[b]		
½ cup (75g)	kamut	free	lemons		
½ cup (75g)	millet	free	limes		
1 cup (150g)	oatmeal	1 cup (150g)	loganberries[c]		
½ cup (75g)	quinoa	½	mango		
½ cup (75g)	rye	2	nectarines (small)		
½ cup (75g)	spelt	1	orange (large)		
½ cup (75g)	SWG** cereal	½	papaya (large)		
½ cup (75g)	raw granola	1	peach (medium)		
	Fruits*	1	pear (medium)		
1	apple (medium)	2	persimmons		
4	apricots (small)	1 cup (150g)	pineapple		
½	banana (medium)	2	plums (small)		
1 cup (150g)	blackberries	1	pomegranate (small)		
1 cup (150g)	blueberries	4	prunes (small)		
1 cup (150g)	boysenberries	¼ cup (60g)	Raisins		
1 cup (150g)	cantaloupe	1 cup (150g)	raspberries		

Notes: *Serving sizes of grains and legumes are measured cooked; those of fruits and vegetables are measured raw.

**SWG = sprouted whole grain (e.g., Ezekiel 4:9 products).

Free = Use as needed for seasoning.

[a] Japanese radish.

[b] Similar to an orange but small like a grape.

[c] Cross between a blackberry and raspberry.

[d] Any but iceberg.

[e] Similar to a turnip.

[f] Orange-fleshed squashes (e.g., acorn, butternut, and kabocha).

[g] Similar to a cantaloupe.

Mixed Types: Carbohydrate Choices

Serving	Legumes*	Serving	Low-Starch Veg*	Serving	Low-Starch Veg*
½ cup (75g)	adzuki beans	1	artichoke	½ cup (75g)	turnip
½ cup (75g)	black beans	1 cup (150g)	asparagus	1 cup (150g)	zucchini
½ cup (75g)	black-eyed beans	½ cup (75g)	bamboo shoots		
½ cup (75g)	fava beans	1 cup (150g)	bok choy		
½ cup (75g)	garbanzo beans	1 cup (150g)	broccoli		
½ cup (75g)	great Northern beans	1 cup (150g)	brussels sprouts		
½ cup (75g)	green beans	1 cup (150g)	cabbage		
½ cup (75g)	green peas	1 cup (150g)	cauliflower		
½ cup (75g)	lentils	1 cup (150g)	celery		
½ cup (75g)	lima beans	1 cup (150g)	cucumber		
½ cup (75g)	mung beans	1 cup (150g)	daikon[a]		
½ cup (75g)	navy beans	1 cup (150g)	eggplant		
½ cup (75g)	pink beans	1 cup (150g)	fennel		
½ cup (75g)	pinto beans	free	garlic		
½ cup (75g)	red beans	free	gingerroot		
½ cup (75g)	white beans	1 cup (150g)	jicama		
	High-Starch Veg*	1 cup (150g)	kale		
1 cup (150g)	beets	free	lettuce[d]		
1 cup (150g)	carrots	1 cup (150g)	mushrooms		
½ cup (75g)	Jerusalem artichoke	1 cup (150g)	okra		
½ cup (75g)	parsnips	5	olives		
½ cup (75g)	potato (white)	1	onion (medium)		
½ cup (75g)	potato (sweet)	1 cup (150g)	pepper (bell)		
¼ cup (60g)	water chestnuts	free	pepper (hot)		
	Dairy	½ cup (75g)	pumpkin		
½ cup (75g)	milk (raw)	½ cup (75g)	radishes		
6 oz (168g)	plain yogurt	½ cup (75g)	rutabaga[e]		
		1 cup (150g)	salad greens[d]		
		1 cup (150g)	spinach		
		½ cup (75g)	squash (winter)[f]		

Notes: *Serving sizes of grains and legumes are measured cooked; those of fruits and vegetables are measured raw.

**SWG = sprouted whole grain (e.g., Ezekiel 4:9 products).

Free = Use as needed for seasoning.

[a] Japanese radish.

[b] Similar to an orange but small like a grape.

[c] Cross between a blackberry and raspberry.

[d] Any but iceberg.

[e] Similar to a turnip.

[f] Orange-fleshed squashes (e.g., acorn, butternut, and kabocha).

[g] Similar to a cantaloupe.

Fat Choices: All Metabolism Types

Fat Choices

Serving	Fat
1 tsp	olive oil
1 tsp	fish oil
1 tsp	cod liver oil
1 tsp	flax seed oil
1 tsp	raw butter
1 oz	avocado[a]
free[b]	coconut oil
1 oz	raw cheese

Note: The fat content of fattier foods such as eggs, meats, oily fish, and nuts has been accounted for in the allotted servings and calories for each metabolism type, so no separate fat servings need to be counted for these foods.

[a] Avocado is a fruit. Protein Types also may use it as a carbohydrate choice (2 ounces).

[b] The Program does not limit the amount of coconut oil that you can consume each day or account for it in the Sample Meal Plans, Done for You Meal Plans and Allowable Servings Guide. A reasonable amount would be 1–2 tsp three times per day for cooking.

*Mixed Types – Remember you are using both the Protein Type choices charts and the Carb Type choices chart for your food choices.

Good, Better, Best

	Good	Better	Best!
Meat	Hormone-free, antibiotic free	Organic, hormone-free, antibiotic free	Organic free-range, grass-fed, hormone-free, antibiotic free
Dairy	Hormone-free, antibiotic free	Organic, hormone-free, antibiotic free	Raw, certified organic (or avoid altogether)
Eggs	Whole, organic eggs	Whole, organic eggs rich in Omega-3s	Whole, grass-fed, free-range eggs (from a local farm)
Bread	Whole grain breads	Spelt bread, rice bread	Sprouted Whole Grain (SWG) bread
Grains	No white/enriched grains	No wheat. Choose spelt or rye instead	No gluten. Choose grains like quinoa, oats (make sure they're gluten free), and brown/wild rice.
Produce	Incorporate fresh fruits and vegetables into your daily meal plans	Purchase organic fruits and vegetables from the list of produce that has been shown to have the highest levels of pesticide residue in the shopping section.	Check out your local farmers' markets for non-synthetically pesticide grown local produce. If shopping at the grocery store, purchase all organic produce.
Seafood	Canned wild-caught seafood	Frozen wild-caught seafood	Fresh wild-caught seafood

	Good	Better	Best!
Sweeteners	Truvia, Stevia products that may contain traces of maltodextrin. Xylitol: completely natural, but does have the potential to cause stomach discomfort	Raw honey and pure maple syrup: healthy choices but should be used in moderation.	Stevia: almost free of calories, doesn't trigger a rise in blood sugar.
Alcohol	Limit alcohol consumption. A good alcohol option is vodka on the rocks; fruit juice only adds empty sugar calories. The best brand is Chopin, which is made from potatoes, not wheat.	Keep alcohol intake to 1-3 glasses per week. A better alcohol option is organic red wine. The rice flavor encourages you to drink slowly. Red wine also contains fewer calories and carbohydrates than other types of alcohol.	Cut out alcohol completely
Flours	Whole wheat flour: better choices than all-purpose flour.	Spelt flour, oat flour, millet flour.	Almond flour, coconut flour, rice flour. With the popularity of many people going "gluten free" there is no shortage of recipes you can find using these delicious flours. They are also very readily available to purchase at most supermarkets and can also be found online.

	Good	Better	Best!
Snacks	Organic "snack foods," store-bought trail mix	Lara bars, Luna bars	Make your own! Visit the Recipes section of beyonddiet.com for ideas! http://www.beyonddiet.com/recipes
Restaurants	Follow the guidelines set out in this article:	Eat at organic restaurants (still following the guidelines for Good eating). Use this guide to help you find ones near you: eatwellguide.com	Keep eating out to a minimum (save it for cheat days). There are so many delicious recipes on Beyond Diet, you'll feel like you're eating out anyway.
Condiments	Organic condiments	Organic, sugar-free, store-bought condiments	Make your own! There are recipes on the site for ketchup, mustard, BBQ sauce, mayonnaise, and many more!
Beverages	Tea and organic coffee. However, you need to increase your water intake to compensate for these.	Herbal teas - No need to increase your water intake to compensate for these.	WATER! Add lemon/lime (or other fruit) and/or a little stevia to your water to give it a little more taste.
Caffeine	Zevia (soda made with stevia)	Organic coffee	Wu-Long tea, Green tea http://go.beyonddiet.com/wulongshopping

	Good	Better	Best!
Supplements	Omega-3 (derived from wild fish). Call the company for details on their fish.	Omega-3 (derived from wild fish). Greens product (make sure it is gluten, soy, and sugar free)	BioTrust OmegaKrill 5X. Athletic Greens.
Dressings	Store-bought olive oil-based dressings with no added sugar (ex. Neuman's Organics)	Olive oil and vinegar	Make your own!
Exercise	Make small changes in your day that will get you to move: Take the stairs instead of the elevator. Park your car far from the entrance to any store.	Incorporate a walk/swim/bike rie into your day a couple times a week.	Work out 3-4 times a week. Include cardio and strength exercises. Use Isabel's Fast Five Exercise.

The Quick Start Guide

Congratulations on your decision to live a healthier life. I am so excited to be on this wonderful journey alongside you.

Now that you have this program, you will see all the wonderful information Beyond Diet has to offer. In order to ensure your success, I highly recommend you follow the steps to following this program as I have outlined for you (if you are reading this Quick Start Guide first, you are in the right place).

Reading this Quick Start Guide is your first steps to success. I have made each topic easy to read and simple to understand. Don't worry. We will go into each topic in more depth later in the program, but right now all you need to do is read through the Quick Start Guide and then I will tell you where to go next. Sound like a plan?

You will see that there are many eye opening topics and principles presented in this program. They are the exact principles that have helped thousands of people lose weight and make a permanent change in their lives.

As with any new change in your life, you may have some questions or just need a little extra help along the way. That is why we have created the Beyond Diet community.

Are you ready to get started? Let's jump right in!

A journey of a thousand miles begins with a single step.
Start now!

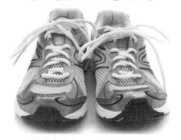

The Facts...Get ready to feel awesome!

Below are the simple facts you need to know in order to successfully begin the first set of Beyond Diet Meal Plans. Just knowing these facts will arm you with a wealth of knowledge to be successful in the first few weeks. Each topic will be covered in more depth later in the program, but for now, this is the perfect place to start.

1. Set up your mind for success.

The first principle we're going to cover has nothing to do with food at all, but has everything to do with your health and your success on this program. What many people don't realize is that the thoughts they think each day can affect their weight loss dramatically.

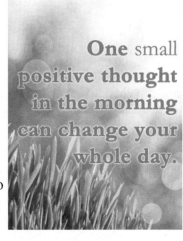

One small **positive thought** in the morning **can change your** whole day.

Consider this...

Let's say Sally and Joe both start the Beyond Diet program on the same day. Sally goes into the program with the mind set, "This is going to be great. I can already see my new body coming!" Joe, on the other hand, starts the program, but with the completely opposite mind set, "Oh what's the use? I've tried to lose weight so many other times. I guess I'll just see if I fail at this too."

If you had to guess, which person do you think has a greater chance of reaching their weight loss goals? Yup, Sally. Because she started off in the right mind set.

I'm asking you to do the same. I'm asking you to start this program with an open mind and to know that you too can be as successful as thousands of other people who have lost weight using these methods.

Spend some time today thinking and writing down exactly what you want for your health, your weight and your life. See yourself in the healthy, beautiful body you've always dreamed about and believe it is possible for you.

(If you haven't done so already, please be sure to add your visualization at the top of your profile page. I'm excited to read it).

2. Let's kick sugar once and for all!

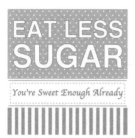

It is no longer a secret or even a shock to most people that refined sugar causes weight gain and is one of the leading causes of obesity in the world. Sugar is also extremely addictive (causing feelings of highs and lows in the body similar to most drugs). And the negative side effects are just as bad as drugs, if not worse.

Americans, truly, don't realize how much sugar they are consuming in one day. Most soft drinks, juices and even some "health" drinks have anywhere between 5-10 teaspoons [25-50 mL] of sugar in each 8 ox [236 mL] serving. Can you imagine putting 8 oz [236 mL] of water in a cup, adding 10 teaspoons [50 mL] of white sugar, and then drinking it? Well this is exactly what you are doing when you drink any kind of soft drink, juice and most other drinks on the market today.

And it's not just drinks that are loaded with sugar. Most cereals and packaged foods have sugar (or some form of sugar) listed as the first or second ingredient (which means it is the ingredient in the highest quantity). The following words on a nutritional label mean "sugar" and should probably be avoided:

- Corn Sweetener, Corn Syrup, or Corn Syrup Solids, Dehydrated Cane Juice, Dextrin, Dextrose, Fructose, Fruit Juice Concentrate, Glucose, High Fructose Corn Syrup, Lactose, Maltodextrin, Malt Syrup, Maltose, Raw Sugar, Rice Syrup, Saccharose, Sucrose, Syrup, Treacle, Turbinado Sugar, Xylose

Fortunately for those looking for a lean, defined body, once you stop eating sugar, your addiction will quickly disappear. People who are "on" sugar crave it all the time. People who are "off" sugar don't even miss it. Weaning yourself off sugar and sugar containing products will cause a drastic and immediate change in your weight. The first few days may be a bit of a "detox" (just like a drug) but these symptoms quickly disappear (and so do the pounds!)

3. Artificial Sweeteners are NOT a good replacement to sugar.

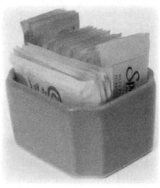

Many times when people decide to give up sugar, they quickly resort to artificial sweeteners. Artificial sweeteners are definitely not the answer! Sorbitol, saccharin, aspartame and sucralose are actually worse for you than sugar itself. All of these artificial sweeteners have been linked to cancer, tumors, and obesity. Yes, artificial sweeteners cause weight gain by disrupting your body's natural hormones. Studies have shown that when people give up their daily "Diet Drink" (filled with aspartame) they quickly lose up to 10 pounds [4.5 kilos] just by eliminating the consumption of this toxic sweetener.

So it is equally important to eliminate any food that contains the above mentioned sweeteners as it is to eliminate sugar from your daily intake.

Most people's next question is then, "Well what is left if I want something sweet?" A great alternative to sugar and artificial sweeteners is the supplement STEVIA. Stevia is a naturally sweet plant native to Paraguay that is 30 times sweeter than sugar in its unprocessed form. With hundreds of studies showing stevia is a safe alternative, it's the next big thing. No wonder. It's all-natural, contains zero calories, and has a zero glycemic index. Stevia leaves are 250-400 times sweeter than sugar and perfect for helping anyone wean themselves away from refined white sugar and artificial sweeteners. Stevia products are great for beverages, soft foods, and baking. Stevia products are available in most local natural foods and health food stores. In grocery stores, Stevia products are typically found in the health food aisle with other supplements.

4. Let's go back to eating "real food."

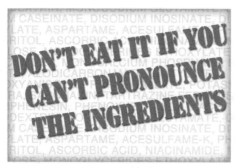

Have you noticed how much fatter Americans have gotten since more "weight loss" and "diet" foods have been put out on the market? Well, I assure you it's no coincidence. Processed foods can truly be considered "Non Foods" since they resemble more of a science experiment than they do real food.

To make differentiating between healthy natural food vs. non-foods easy, just stay away from anything that contains ingredients on a label that you can't pronounce. If the ingredients list to your favorite cereal is more complicated than your college organic chemistry final, chances are you should stay away from it at all costs. These chemicals are all toxins to your body (just as artificial sweeteners are) and your liver becomes extremely overwhelmed trying to rid your body of these harmful toxins. Why is this important in your efforts to lose fat? Well, the other job of your liver is to burn body fat and if it is too busy ridding you of toxic overload, it has no time (or energy) to get rid of your unwanted fat.

5. Eat the "right carbs" for optimal health and fat loss.

I do agree that reducing the amount of carbohydrates in your meal plans will help you lose weight and lean down. But you must reduce the bad and increase the good. Eating fibrous carbohydrates like fruits and vegetables actually turns your body into a fat burning machine. Eating starchy carbs like rice and potatoes after a workout will also help you develop the lean, muscular physique most men and women are looking for. It is the processed and refined wheat and grains that are causing everyone to feel bloated and have a difficult time

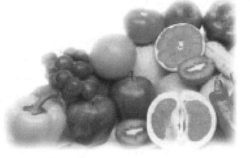

losing weight.

Don't fall into the "no carb" trap. Learn the right carb approach to look great and feel great.

6. Fire up your metabolism by eating regularly (don't eat like a sumo wrestler!)

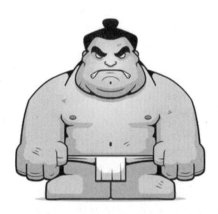

Sumo wrestlers make a concerted effort to get fat for their sport. So if your number one goal was to GET FAT this is exactly what you could do:

1. Skip breakfast and eat very little all day long.

2. Eat the bulk of your caloric intake in a large heavy meal, filled with complex carbohydrates in the evening.

3. Go to bed after eating this heavy meal.

That's it. This strategy has been working for sumo wrestlers for years. And you know who else it is working for? The 130 million Americans who are overweight or obese.

You must develop the habit of eating frequent meals all day long to develop the kind of warp speed metabolism that is going to allow you to get lean and stay lean (no sense in getting there without being able to maintain it right?) Eat 4-6 well portioned meals each day and you will see your body burn fat faster than you can say "sumo wrestler."

7. Water, it does a body good.

If you often feel like you are starving all day no matter how much food you've consumed, chances are you may be severely dehydrated. Many people actually mistake dehydration for hunger and eat tons more calories than they actually need when all they really needed to do was drink some water!

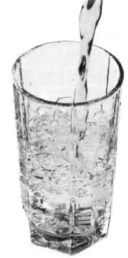

It would be impossible to pick up any diet or weight loss book without it saying somewhere "drink 8-10 cups of water each day." Even if all health and nutrition gurus don't agree on all the same principles, they do all agree on one: water is the magic potion to ensure weight loss. When you consider that water helps the body metabolize stored fat, rid the body of waste (as in unwanted fats and toxins), and is a natural diuretic and a natural laxative, no wonder it is an absolute MUST when fat loss is your goal. Drink a minimum of 1/2 of your body weight in ounces of filtered water each day to ensure that your body rids itself of the unwanted fat you are aiming to lose.

8. Throw out all those deceiving "Health Foods."

Yes, you have been scammed. You and approximately hundreds of thousands of other people who have purchased pre-packaged "health" foods. There are many health foods on the market today that are causing people to gain weight, as well as making it near impossible for them to lose weight. Have you ever purchased the foods that someone claimed to be "guaranteed to make you lose weight" only to see the scale go up instead of down? Frustrated dieters all over the world can't figure out why their new weight loss shake is not working like the commercial suggested. Well, one of the nasty culprits causing millions of people to pack on the pounds is hydrogenated oil. There are thousands of health foods that contain this toxic oil. Weight Watchers and Lean Cuisine meals and bars almost all contain hydrogenated oil (and they are supposed to be good for you?). Even some energy sports bars and shakes are loaded up with hydrogenated oils and many other toxic preservatives.

Another nasty culprit is processed soy. This is always a shock to most people (especially die hard vegetarians) who have been falsely led to believe that soy is actually good for you. Well if you lived in Asia you would quickly see that most Asians eat soy in small quantities in the form of old fashioned fermented soy (such as miso, tempeh, natto, shoyu, and tamari) not the processed, toxic soy that is used in so many vegetarian type products and weight loss products on the market today. The worst of today's soy protein products are soy protein isolate, soy protein concentrate, texturized vegetable protein and hydrolyzed vegetable protein. These ingredients are found in everything from shake powders, energy bars and veggie burgers to canned tuna. The worst soy oil products are margarines and shortenings made from partially hydrogenated soybean oil containing dangerous trans fatty acids. So avoid these forms of toxic soy at all costs. Not only will you be saving yourself from a myriad of

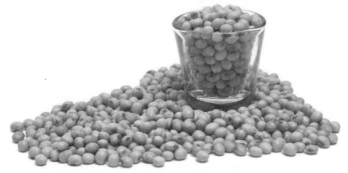

health problems (like decreased thyroid function and hormone disruption) you will also see a dramatic loss in unwanted body fat.

9. Learn to love fat... I mean the *right kind* of FAT.

While some thought Atkins was the best thing since sliced bread, others

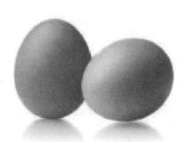

thought that fat was the root of all evil. This is only partially true and the complete elimination of all fats from your diet is a BIG mistake. Yes, you should eliminate unhealthy fats like hydrogenated oils (sorry, that means no French fries or doughnuts). But the healthy fats found in wild fish and nuts are absolutely necessary for you body to function at optimum. These fats, called Omega 3 essential fatty acids, are actually so critical to your body's functioning, that it is very difficult to experience any weight loss without including them in your meal plan.

Where do you find these Omega 3's? You find them in salmon, walnuts, chia seeds and organic eggs. Make these foods an integral part of your eating regimen and you will see some great results in your weight loss efforts. A high quality Omega 3 supplement also works wonders for your body and helps to burn off unwanted fat. Take a few capsules with each meal to ensure you are getting your Omega 3's daily.

10. Build your body and stop hunger by eating Protein.

Protein is not just for bodybuilders. It's for every person who wants to achieve a lean, slender and toned physique. (Did I just describe every person on the planet?) Protein not only fuels your muscles, it also helps stabilize your blood sugar and prevents hunger. So you get the benefit of lean, toned muscles and a way to 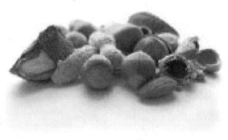 NOT be hungry. Sounds like a win, win to me. Unfortunately, most people go the entire day without eating any protein at all. It's no wonder these are the same people that complain of a flabby body, fatigue, and hunger pangs that just won't go away. Include a source of healthy protein into each meal (that includes snacks). Wonderful sources of protein are grass fed meats, free range poultry, organic eggs, wild fish, and organic raw nuts.

Important Facts

1. Cola is worse than you think.

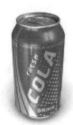

Soda is absolutely toxic for your body. Just look at the ingredients label of a can of soda. One of the first two ingredients is likely high fructose corn syrup, an ingredient that should be avoided at all costs. While most people are aware of the dangers of drinking regular soda, many people falsely believe that "diet" soda is in some way a good thing for losing body fat when, in fact, there is absolutely nothing healthy about drinking diet soda. Diet soda tricks your sweet tooth into thinking you're getting something for nothing, which can actually lead to overeating. Worse yet, drinking soda is associated with obesity, diabetes, heart disease, liver damage, high blood pressure, osteoporosis, even some cancers.

2. Did you know salt is good for you?

You don't need to cut salt out completely, but you do need to change the type of salt you use. Salt has such a bad reputation because 99% of the world's salt research has been done on commercial table salt.

Instead of refined table salt, use unrefined sea salt or Himalayan rock salt. These slats are extremely healthy and have the exact opposite effect of refined salt. They provide sodium chloride in a form that the body needs to function and offer the perfect balance of minerals, nutrients, and sodium chloride that the body needs for optimum health.

3. Eating the right kind of bread is critical to weight loss success.

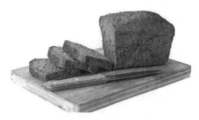

Bread is a staple of the American diet. Unfortunately, most of us eat the absolute worst kind of bread: the kind made from refined grains. White bread is stripped of essential vitamins and nutrients during processing, and the whole wheat bread the American public has been led to believe is healthy contains processed wheat, which is deficient in nutrients. If you are not willing to forgo eating bread altogether, I suggest you look into stocking your fridge with sprouted whole grain (SWG) bread.

4. Cook with butter or coconut oil.

Fake butters are made from unhealthy, unnatural ingredients which are perceived as toxins in the body. As I've mentioned, it is your liver's job to filter these unnatural ingredients out of your bloodstream. The more work your liver as to do, the harder it is to maintain a healthy weight. Replace those fake butters with raw, organic butter. This is actually one of the healthiest whole foods you can include in your diet.

Another great oil to incorporate into your eating plan every day is unrefined coconut oil. Besides the fact that it tastes amazing, it has been called a "miracle" food by physicians and health professionals for its ability ot speed up the metabolism and help the body burn off unwanted fat.

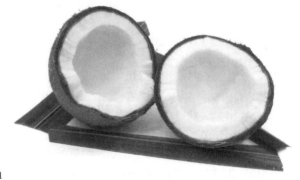

5. No more canola oil.

When answering the question "is canola oil bad for you," most people ahve focused on the fact that canola oil was, originally, a derivative of rapeseed oil. Rapeseed oil, beyond having the kind of name that makes you want to stay away, contains high levels of **erucic acid**, which is associated with heart disease. In the past several decades, farmers and researchers selectively bred rapeseed in order to lower the amount of erucic acid found in the oils.

But even if you don't have to worry that you're cooking your heart healthy meals in an oil that may cause heart disease, the larger – and unavoidable – problem with canola oil cannot be ignored.

Most seeds used to make canola oil in the United States are *genetically modified*. Canola seeds are planted in massive fields, and nearly 80% of those seeds have been genetically modified so farmers can spray their fields with weed killers without also killing the crops. So using canola oil means putting something in your body that has been modified to withstand industrial pesticides.

Canola oil is heavily processed. After being extracted from the seeds, canola oil is chemically refined, bleached with organic acids, and deodorized, so the oil you use to cook will neither look nor smell as it does naturally.

Polyunsaturated fats oxidize under high heat. Oxidization can occur either during processing or cooking. The oxidization of polyunsaturated fats releases free radicals into the body, increasing your risk for many diseases, including cancer.

Wow!

Did you learn a lot? I hope you did. Because it is my #1 goal to give you all of the information you need to not only drop your unwanted fat for good, but also make you feel great every single day.

Right around this point is where people ask me, "Isabel, now what do you want me to do with all of this information?"

Lucky for you I have figured out a way to make this as easy for you as possible (not to mention showing you incredible results in the least amount of time).

I have created for you very easy to follow meal plans that you will be using for the next 14 days. These meal plans will help you to apply the principles you just learned, without having to figure any of this out yourself. I've done all the work for you.

Sound good?

So your next step is to open up the 14 Day Meal Plans and all the instructions you need are there.

But before you go... I have a few more items to let you know about:

Because I know any lifestyle change can bring up a lot of questions, we have set up the Beyond Diet website so you always have a place to get all of your questions answered and to share your successes along the way. I want you to know...

We are here for you! Please remember that. I do not want you to ever feel like you are in this alone. That is why we have created the ASK and SHARE sections in Beyond Diet.

Please ASK Us

If you have a specific question about following the meal plans or any of the information you have just read, please ask it in the ASK section (you can find the ASK section on the homepage of your members area). You will see that once you start typing your question, some suggested answers will come up. Your specific question may have already been answered on the site, or you can post a new one.

Please SHARE With Us

If you would like to share any detail about your life or your health journey, please share it with our loving community in the SHARE section (you can also find the SHARE section on the home page of your members area). You will see what a true family we are in Beyond Diet and how encouraging and helpful everyone is. We love to hear your successes as well as any challenges that may come up along the way. Please post those in the SHARE section. I look forward to reading it.

14 Days of Supercharged Meal Plans

www.BeyondDiet.com

Introduction

I'm so excited for you to get started on these meal plans. In a few days from today you are already going to see a big difference in how you feel and how you look.

These meal plans were created to help you easily implement all of the information you learned in the Quick Start Guide. Please be sure to read the instructions, the shopping list, the meal plans and the FAQs section before you begin.

How to Use These Meal Plans

There are 12 meal plans for you to follow. You will follow the meal plans for 6 days and then give yourself a "cheat day" (more details on that below). You will then follow the meal plans for another 6 days and then give yourself another cheat day on Day 14.

Please take some time now to look through the shopping list and the meal plans and some general questions I have answered for you below.

Grocery Shopping Guide

Week 1 - Days 1 through 6
(*Some products purchased during week 1 will be left over to use for week 2)

Produce	Amount	Notes	Buy Online - Recommended Items
Romaine Lettuce	3 pack		*Online shopping not recommended for perishable items
Spinach	1 package	4 cups	
Tomato	7	medium	
Cucumber	3	medium	
Peppers	4	medium	
Celery	8	large stalks	
Carrots	4-6	large	
Onion	1	medium	
Green Beans	1/2 cup		
Broccoli	3 cups		
Cauliflower	1 cup		
Sweet Potato	1	medium	
Spaghetti Squash	1	small	
Baby Carrots	2 cups		
Zucchini	1	medium	
Avocado	6 oz	about 2 avocados	
Apple (green)	2	small	
Banana	1	medium	
Lemon	2	medium to large	

Meat & Seafood	Amount	Notes	Buy Online - Recommended Items
Chicken Breast	9 oz		
Chicken (dark)	14 oz		
Chicken Sausage	6 oz		
Bacon	6 slices	Pork or Turkey	
Ground Turkey	12 oz		
Sliced Turkey	4 oz		
Ground Buffalo	4 oz		
Canned Tuna	4 oz		
Salmon	4 oz		
Shrimp	4 oz		
Tilapia	5 oz		
Dairy	**Amount**	**Notes**	**Buy Online - Recommended Items**
Eggs	2 dozen		
Nuts, Seeds, Butters and Beans	**Amount**	**Notes**	**Buy Online - Recommended Items**
Raw Almonds	2 oz		
Raw Walnuts	2 oz		
Raw Macadamia Nuts	1 oz		
Raw Brazil Nuts	1/2 oz		
Raw Pumpkin Seeds	1 1/2 oz		
Breads and Grains	**Amount**	**Notes**	**Buy Online - Recommended Items**
Sprouted Whole Grain Bread	1 small loaf	Ezekiel 4:9	
Rice Cereal	2 cups		
Oatmeal	2 cups	Dry	

Condiments & Other	Amount	Notes	Buy Online - Recommended Items
Coconut Oil	1		
Extra Virgin Olive Oil	1		
Vinegar	1		
Soy Sauce	1	Wheat Free	
Dijon Mustard	1		
Garlic Powder	1		
Cinnamon	1		
Unrefined Sea Salt	1		http://go.beyonddiet.com/ aztecseasalt
Protein Powder	1		http://go.beyonddiet.com/ biotrustproteinpowder

Week 2 - Days 8 through 13

Produce	Amount	Notes	Buy Online - Recommended Items
Romaine Lettuce	3 pack		
Spinach	1 package	4 cups	
Tomato	6	medium	
Cucumber	3	medium	
Peppers	4	medium	
Celery	8	large stalks	
Carrots	4-6	large	
Onion	1	medium	
Green Beans	1/2 cup		
Green Peas	1/2 cup		
Broccoli	3 cups		
Cauliflower	2 cups		
Spaghetti Squash	1	small	
Zucchini	1	medium	
Avocado	6 oz	about 2 avocados	
Apple (green)	6	medium	
Banana	2	medium	
Strawberries	1 small package	1 cup	
Lemon	2	medium to large	

14 Days of Supercharged Meal Plans - Grocery Shopping Guide

Meat & Seafood	Amount	Notes	Buy Online - Recommended Items
Chicken Breast	9 oz		
Chicken (dark)	12 oz		
Bacon	6 slices	Pork or Turkey	
Ground Turkey	12 oz		
Sliced Turkey	8 oz		
Ground Buffalo	4 oz		
Canned Tuna	4 oz		
Salmon	4 oz		
Scallops	4 oz		
Tilapia	5 oz		

Recipes

Turkey Chili
*This recipe makes 4 servings, so remember to divide it into 4 to get your 1 serving.

Ingredients
2 tsp butter, divided
1 lb lean ground turkey
To taste salt and freshly ground black pepper
1 cup coarsely chopped red bell pepper
1 medium onion, coarsely chopped (~3/4 cup)
2/3 cup coarsely chopped celery (~2/3 stalk)
1 clove garlic, minced
2 tsp chili powder
1 tsp paprika
1 tsp ground cumin
1/8 tsp ground cayenne pepper
14 1/2 oz plum tomatoes, chopped (canned with juice is fine)
1/2 cup chicken stock (or low-fat low-sodium chicken broth)
1 bay leaf

Directions
Heat 1 tsp butter in a 3-quart saucepan over high heat. Add the turkey, and season to taste with the salt and black pepper. Break up the turkey and cook for 2-3 minutes, or until browned. Remove to a bowl and cover to keep warm. Reduce the heat to low, heat the other 1 tsp butter, and cook the red pepper, onion, celery, and garlic for 3-5 minutes, or until vegetables begin to soften. Add the chili powder, paprika, cumin, and cayenne and cook, stirring, for 1 minute. Increase the heat to medium, and add the tomatoes, stock, and bay leaf. Bring to a boil over high heat. Reduce the heat to medium-low, and simmer uncovered for 15 minutes.

Add the browned turkey, and simmer 5 minutes more. Remove and discard the bay leaf before serving.

Isabel's Famous Salad Dressing

Ingredients
1 tsp organic yellow mustard, or Dijon mustard
1/2 tsp garlic powder
1/2 tsp Celtic sea salt
1/4 cup apple cider vinegar
3/4 cup organic extra virgin olive oil
2 Tbsp raw parmesan cheese, grated (optional)

Directions
Combine all ingredients in a salad shaker, and shake well!

The apple cider vinegar is the "magic ingredient," but the olive oil is the main ingredient and will make up most of the dressing. Enjoy!

Frequently Asked Questions

What if there is a meal or a food I don't like?

I understand that each of us has different tastes and that some of these meals may taste great to you while some may not appeal to you at all. You can easily adjust your meals for the day by choosing the breakfasts you like, the snack you like...etc...and mix and match them to create your own meal plans. Each meal is interchangeable. Just don't exchange a breakfast with a lunch or a lunch with a dinner. You can only exchange the same type of meal (breakfast with breakfast, lunch with lunch.

Do I need to modify these meal plans based on my weight?

The meal plans are roughly based on a 1600 calorie meal plan. I have found that 1600 calories of the right food combinations is sufficient to keep most people from being hungry while simultaneously quickly burning off a lot of body fat.

If you have been a dieter for a long time and 1600 sounds a bit high to you, I assure you it's not. Restricting calories to low levels can be damaging to your metabolism and make your body hold on to fat instead of burning it off. Also, the foods that I have chosen in these meal plans are foods that will naturally stimulate fat burning in your body.

If you feel like you need more food, and are hungry while following these plans, you can begin by increasing the protein serving by 1 ounce at a time. For example, if lunch calls for 4 oz salmon, increase it to 5 or 6 if necessary.

Remember, also, that these meal plans are to be followed for 2 weeks. You will then be creating new meal plans for yourself that are specific to your own personal needs.

What can I drink while following these meal plans?

1. Water - 1/2 of your body weight in ounces of water each day (e.g. if you weigh 150 lbs., then 75 oz of water throughout the course of each

day)

2. Green Tea - (careful with the caffeine content) sweetened with stevia or xylitol

3. Coffee - (1 cup per day maximum) sweetened with stevia or xylitol (no milk or creamer)

What can I eat on my cheat days?

You can eat whatever you like without gorging yourself. Don't eat until you are overly full at each meal. You can eat whatever foods you would until you are satisfied, just be reasonable. Two slices of pizza is a meal, but a whole pie is not! A slice of cake is a great dessert, not the whole cake! (I think you get the point.)

What I do on my cheat days is just eat as I feel like it all day. I don't plan like I would on all my other days and I eat whatever I am craving. For example, I may wake up and make pancakes, have sushi for lunch followed by some cookies, and go out to dinner and choose whatever appeals to me on the menu (including dessert). As you can see, I do not eat with reckless abandon, but I don't plan my healthy meals like I do on the other days of the week.

How much weight should I expect to lose with these meal plans?

You can expect to lose anywhere between 5-10 pounds in these first 2 weeks... some people may lose more, some people may lose less. Please do not focus so much on the number on the scale, but focus more on how you feel, how your clothes are fitting and the wonderful habits you are changing in these first 2 weeks.

What should I do when I complete these 14 days?

Return to "Start Here" on Beyonddiet.com and go on to Step 3.

Week 1 Cooking Suggestions & Tips

The following ideas are just suggestions and how I put together my own meals each day. As long as you stay within your serving sizes and use the foods listed, you can put these meals together however is best for you. Remember these are only suggestions.

Below I have explained how I would prepare the meals that are listed in the meal plans provided. I did not include every meal, as some are self explanatory.

Day 1

Breakfast
I would cook the spinach using coconut oil and then add in the eggs to make a spinach omelet. I would then eat it over the sliced tomato.

Lunch
I would broil the salmon seasoned with salt and pepper. I would most likely have done this the night before to have it ready for the next day's lunch. I would have it cold over the salad and use olive oil and lemons as my salad dressing.

Snack / Post Workout
Looking ahead, tomorrow's dinner calls for chicken legs (dark meat chicken) so I would probably bake a whole chicken and use the breast for my snack / post workout and save some dark meat for the next day. My husband would also eat some so none of it would go to waste.

I would bake the sweet potato in the oven for 45 minutes. I would eat the broccoli raw or lightly steamed.

Dinner
You can use the turkey chili recipe provided on page 159 or make a burger and top with sliced tomatoes. I would then make a salad of romaine lettuce, carrots and celery. (Make sure to make enough for tomorrow's lunch.)

Day 2

Breakfast
I would make "sausage and peppers." First cook the onions and peppers in coconut oil and then add in your sausage.

Lunch
I always like to have my lunch ready the night before and eating leftovers is usually the easiest for me. Lunch will be leftovers from last night.

Snack / Post Workout
Scramble the egg whites and make an egg sandwich (you can use a small amount of coconut oil to cook).

Dinner
I would have a chicken leg leftover from the chicken I made the day before and I would measure out 4 oz of dark meat. Saute the green beans in coconut oil.

Day 3

Snack / Post Workout
Put 2 scoops of Protein Powder, water, ice and a banana in the blender to make a snack / post workout shake.

Dinner
I would use 1 tsp (5 mL) of the coconut oil to cook my turkey burger, 1 tsp to cook the peppers and onions and 1 tsp to cook the spinach.

Day 4

Breakfast
I would cut up the chicken and the avocado and serve that over the cauliflower.

Lunch

I finely chop 1 celery stalk, 1 carrot and a 1/4 red pepper and add that to the tuna fish along with 1 Tbsp (15 mL) of olive oil to make a "no mayo" tuna salad.

Day 5

Lunch

I add garlic powder, oregano, parsley, thyme, salt and pepper to ground buffalo and make meatballs. I cook them in coconut oil. I saute 2 pieces of garlic and then add the cut up tomato. This will serve as your "sauce." Serve over spaghetti squash.

Snack / Post Workout

I add the Protein Powder right into the cereal.

Day 6

Lunch

Hard boil 4 eggs. Use 2 whole eggs and the whites from the other 2. Mash them all up and add 1 Tbsp (15 mL) Dijon Mustard and 1 tsp (5 mL) olive oil. You can also add salt and pepper to taste. This is your egg salad. Make a side salad and add the beans.

Snack / Post Workout

I add the protein powder right into the oatmeal and sprinkle a little cinnamon on top.

Dinner

I buy "wheat free" soy sauce at the health food store for all my Chinese style recipes. If you can't find this kind, regular soy sauce is ok. Use 1-2 tsp (5-10 mL)(a little goes a long way).

Day 1

Food	Protein	Carbs	Fat	Notes
Breakfast				
2 eggs	2	0	0	
1 cup (180 g) cooked spinach	0	1	0	
1 tomato, sliced	0	1	0	
2 tsp coconut oil - use for cooking spinach and eggs or eat raw	0	0	0	
Totals	2	2	0	
Snack				
1 oz (28 g) almonds (20-24)	2	0	0	
Totals	2	0	0	
Lunch				
4 oz (112 g) cooked salmon	4	0	0	
1/2 cup (38 g) chick peas	0	1	0	
1 cup raw vegetables (spinach, cucumbers, celery, peppers) made into a salad with lettuce	0	1	0	
2 tsp (10 mL) extra virgin olive oil and vinegar or lemon to dress the salad	0	0	2	
Totals	4	2	2	
Snack / Post Workout				
4 oz (112 g) chicken breast	4	0	0	
1 cup (100 g) cooked broccoli	0	1	0	
1/2 cup (112 g) sweet potato	0	1	0	
Totals	4	2	0	
Dinner				
4 oz (112 g) ground turkey	4	0	0	
1 cup tomatoes, onions, carrots, celery (can be used to make chili, as toppings for a burger, or as a side salad	0	1	0	
2 tsp (10 mL) extra virgin olive oil + lemon (used as dressing over salad or to cook veggies for chili)	0	0	2	
Totals	4	1	2	
Totals	16	7	4	

Day 2

Food	Protein	Carbs	Fat	Notes
Breakfast				
3 oz (84 g) chicken sausage	3	0	0	
1 cup (100 g) onions and peppers - cooked	0	1	0	
2 tsp (10 mL) coconut oil - use for cooking veggies and sausage or eat raw	0	0	0	
Totals	**3**	**1**	**0**	
Snack				
2 Tbsp (28 g) nut butter	2	0	0	
1 cup (85 g) baby carrots	0	1	0	
Totals	**2**	**1**	**0**	
Lunch				
4 oz (112 g) ground turkey	4	0	0	
1 cup tomatoes, onions, carrots, and celery (can be used to make chili, as toppings for a burger, or as a side salad)	0	1	0	
2 tsp (10 mL) extra virgin olive oil + lemon (used as dressing over salad or to cook veggies for chili)	0	0	2	
Totals	**4**	**1**	**2**	
Snack / Post Workout				
5 egg whites	4	0	0	
1 tomato sliced	0	1	0	
2 slices sprouted whole grain bread	0	2	0	
Totals	**4**	**3**	**0**	
Dinner				
4 oz (112 g) chicken (dark)	4	0	0	
1/2 cup (57 g) green beans	0	1	0	
1 cup tomato and cucumber salad	0	1	0	
2 tsp (10 mL) extra virgin olive oil + lemon (can be used as dressing for salad	0	0	2	
Totals	**4**	**2**	**2**	
Totals	**17**	**8**	**4**	

Day 3

Food	Protein	Carbs	Fat	Notes
Breakfast				
3 slices bacon (pork or turkey)	3	0	0	
1 slice sprouted whole grain bread	0	1	0	
1 tomato, sliced	0	1	0	
Totals	3	2	0	
Snack				
1/2 oz (14 g) macadamia nuts (5-6)	1	0	0	
Totals	1	0	0	
Lunch				
4 oz (112 g) grilled shrimp	4	0	0	
2 oz (57 g) avocado	0	0	2	
1 cup raw vegetables (spinach, cucumber, celery, peppers) made into a salad with lettuce	0	1	0	
2 Tbsp Isabel's Famous Salad Dressing	0	0	2	
1 small green apple	0	1	0	
Totals	4	2	4	
Snack / Post Workout				
2 scoops BioTrust protein powder with water and ice	3	0	0	
1 banana	0	2	0	
Totals	3	2	0	
Dinner				
4 oz (112 g) ground turkey to use for turkey burger	4	0	0	
1 cup peppers and onions	0	1	0	
1 cup (90-180 g) sauteed spinach	0	1	0	
3 tsp (15 mL) coconut oil	0	0	0	
Totals	4	2	0	
Totals	15	8	4	

Day 4

Food	Protein	Carbs	Fat	Notes
Breakfast				
3 oz (84 g) leftover chicken (dark)	3	0	0	
1 cup (100 g) steamed cauliflower	0	1	0	
2 oz (57 g) avocado	0	0	2	
Totals	**3**	**1**	**2**	
Snack				
2 Tbsp (28 g) nut butter	2	0	0	
1 cup baby carrots	0	1	0	
Totals	**3**	**1**	**2**	
Lunch				
4 oz (112 g) canned tuna (dark)	4	0	0	
1 cup celery, carrots, and red peppers	0	1	0	
1/2 cup (38 g) chickpeas	0	1	0	
1 Tbsp (15 mL) extra virgin olive oil	0	0	3	
Totals	**4**	**2**	**3**	
Snack / Post Workout				
4 oz (112 g) sliced turkey (white)	4	0	0	
1 tomato, sliced	0	1	0	
2 slices sprouted whole grain bread (sandwich)	0	2	0	
Totals	**4**	**3**	**0**	
Dinner				
4 oz (112 g) chicken (dark)	4	0	0	
1 cup (100 g) sauteed garlic broccoli	0	1	0	
1 cup raw vegetables (tomatoes, onions, carrots, celery) made into a salad with lettuce	0	1	0	
3 tsp (15 mL) extra virgin olive oil	0	0	3	
Totals	**4**	**2**	**3**	
Totals	**17**	**8**	**8**	

Day 5

Food	Protein	Carbs	Fat	Notes
Breakfast				
3 oz (84 g) leftover chicken (dark)	3	0	0	
1 cup (100 g) sauteed spinach	0	1	0	
2 tsp (10 mL) coconut oil - use for cooking spinach or eat raw	0	0	0	
1 small green apple	0	1	0	
Totals	3	2	0	
Snack				
1/2 oz pumpkin seeds	1	0	0	
Totals	1	0	0	
Lunch				
4 oz (112 g) ground buffalo (made into meatballs)	4	0	0	
sauteed garlic tomatoes (1 whole tomato)	0	1	0	
1 cup (155 g) spaghetti squash	0	2	0	
2 tsp (10 mL) coconut oil - use for cooking tomato or eat raw	0	0	0	
Totals	4	3	0	
Snack / Post Workout				
2 scoops BioTrust Protein Powder	3	0	0	
1 cup (156 g) cooked rice cereal (hot cereal made from rice)	0	1	0	
Totals	3	1	0	
Dinner				
5 oz (142 g) broiled tilapia	5	0	0	
2 oz (57 g) avocado	0	0	2	
1 cup raw vegetables (cucumber, celery, green peppers) made into a salad with lettuce	0	1	0	
3 tsp (15 mL) extra virgin olive oil	0	0	3	
Totals	5	2	5	
Totals	16	8	5	

Day 6

Food	Protein	Carbs	Fat	Notes
Breakfast				
3 slices bacon (pork or turkey)	3	0	0	
1 egg	1	0	0	
1 tomato, sliced	0	1	0	
Totals	4	1	0	
Snack				
1 oz (28 g) raw walnuts (14 halves)	2	0	0	
Totals	2	0	0	
Lunch				
2 whole eggs + 2 egg whites + 1 Tbsp Dijon mustard + 1 tsp olive oil (to make egg salad)	4	0	1	
1 cup raw vegetables (cucumbers, celery, peppers, carrots) made into a salad with lettuce	0	1	0	
1 Tbsp Isabel's Famous Salad Dressing	0	0	1	
1/2 cup (76 g) chickpeas or kidney beans	0	1	0	
Totals	4	2	2	
Snack / Post Workout				
2 scoops BioTrust protein powder with water and ice	3	0	0	
1 cup dry oatmeal (make with water) add cinnamon to taste	0	1	0	
Totals	3	1	0	
Dinner				
5 oz (142 g) cooked chicken breast	5	0	0	
1 cup peppers and zucchini	0	1	0	
1 cup tomato and cucumber salad	0	1	0	
1-2 tsp (10-15 mL) wheat free soy sauce	0	0	0	
3 tsp (5 mL) extra virgin olive oil	0	0	3	
Totals	5	2	3	
Totals	18	6	5	

Day 7

Cheat Day

What can I eat on my cheat days?
You can eat whatever you like without gorging yourself. Don't eat until you are overly full at each meal. You can eat whatever foods you would until you are satisfied, just be reasonable. Two slices of pizza is a meal, but a whole pie is not! A slice of cake is a great dessert, not the whole cake! (I think you get the point).

What I do on my cheat days is just eat as I feel like it all day. I don't plan like I would on all my other days and I eat whatever I am craving. For example, I may wake up and make pancakes, have sushi for lunch followed by some cookies, and go out to dinner and choose whatever appeals to me on the menu (including dessert). As you can see, I do not eat with reckless abandon, but I don't plan my healthy meals like I do on the other days of the week.

Week 2 Cooking Suggestions & Tips

Day 8

Breakfast
I would cook the spinach using coconut oil and then add in the eggs to make a spinach omelet. I would then eat it over the sliced tomato.

Lunch
I would broil the salmon seasoned with salt and pepper. I would most likely have done this the night before to have it ready for the next day's lunch. I would have it cold over the salad and use olive oil and lemons as my salad dressing.

Snack / Post Workout
Looking ahead, tomorrow's dinner calls for chicken legs (dark meat chicken) so I would probably bake a whole chicken and use the breast for my snack / post workout and save some dark meat for the next day. My

husband would also eat some so none of it would go to waste.

I would eat the cauliflower raw or lightly steamed.

Dinner
You can use the turkey chili recipe provided on page 159 or make a burger and top with sliced tomatoes. I would then make a salad of romaine lettuce, carrots and celery. (Make sure to make enough for tomorrow's lunch.)

Day 9

Breakfast
I would make "sausage and peppers." First cook the onions and peppers in coconut oil and then add in your sausage.

Lunch
I always like to have my lunch ready the night before and eating leftovers is usually the easiest for me. Lunch will be leftovers from last night.

Snack / Post Workout
Scramble the egg whites and make an egg sandwich (you can use a small amount of coconut oil to cook).

Dinner
I would have a chicken leg leftover from the chicken I made the day before and I would measure out 4 oz of dark meat. Saute the green beans in coconut oil.

Day 10

Snack / Post Workout
Put 2 scoops of Protein Powder, water, ice and a banana in the blender to make a snack / post workout shake.

Dinner
I would use 1 tsp (5 mL) of the coconut oil to cook my turkey burger, 1 tsp to cook the peppers and onions and 1 tsp to cook the spinach.

Day 11

Breakfast
I would cut up the eggs and the avocado and serve that over the cauliflower.

Lunch
I finely chop 1 celery stalk, 1 carrot and a 1/4 red pepper and add that to the tuna fish along with 1 Tbsp (15 mL) of olive oil to make a "no mayo" tuna salad.

Day 12

Lunch
I add garlic powder, oregano, parsley, thyme, salt and pepper to ground buffalo and make meatballs. I cook them in coconut oil. I saute 2 pieces of garlic and then add the cut up tomato. This will serve as your "sauce."

Snack / Post Workout
I add the Protein Powder right into the cereal.

Day 13

Lunch
Hard boil 4 eggs. Use 2 whole eggs and the whites from the other 2. Mash them all up and add 1 Tbsp (15 mL) Dijon Mustard and 1 tsp (5 mL) olive oil. You can also add salt and pepper to taste. This is your egg salad. Make a side salad and add the green peas to it.

Dinner

I buy "wheat free" soy sauce at the health food store for all my Chinese style recipes. If you can't find this kind, regular soy sauce is ok. Use 1-2 tsp (5-10 mL)(a little goes a long way).

Day 8

Food	Protein	Carbs	Fat	Notes
Breakfast				
2 eggs	2	0	0	
1 cup (180 g) cooked spinach	0	1	0	
1 tomato, sliced	0	1	0	
2 tsp (10 mL) olive oil	0	0	2	
Totals	2	2	2	
Snack				
1 oz (28 g) almonds (20-24)	2	0	0	
Totals	2	0	0	
Lunch				
4 oz (112 g) cooked salmon	4	0	0	
1/2 cup (38 g) chick peas	0	1	0	
1 cup raw vegetables (lettuce, cucumbers, celery, peppers, carrots) made into a salad	0	1	0	
1 Tbsp (15 mL) Isabel's Famous Salad Dressing	0	0	1	
Totals	4	2	2	
Snack / Post Workout				
4 oz (112 g) chicken breast	4	0	0	
1 cup (90 g) cauliflower	0	1	0	
1 small green apple	0	1	0	
Totals	4	2	0	
Dinner				
4 oz (112 g) ground turkey	4	0	0	
1 cup tomatoes, onions, carrots, celery (can be used to make chili, as toppings for a burger, or as a side salad	0	1	0	
2 tsp (10 mL) extra virgin olive oil + lemon (used as dressing over salad or to cook veggies for chili)	0	0	2	
Totals	4	1	2	
Totals	16	7	5	

Day 9

Food	Protein	Carbs	Fat	Notes
Breakfast				
3 oz (84 g) chicken sausage	3	0	0	
1 cup (100 g) onions and peppers - cooked	0	1	0	
2 tsp (10 mL) coconut oil - use for cooking veggies and sausage or eat raw	0	0	0	
Totals	3	1	0	
Snack				
2 Tbsp (28 g) nut butter	2	0	0	
1 cup (85 g) baby carrots	0	1	0	
Totals	2	1	0	
Lunch				
4 oz (112 g) ground turkey	4	0	0	
1 cup tomatoes, onions, carrots, and celery (can be used to make chili, as toppings for a burger, or as a side salad)	0	1	0	
2 tsp (10 mL) extra virgin olive oil + lemon (used as dressing over salad or to cook veggies for chili)	0	0	2	
Totals	4	1	2	
Snack / Post Workout				
5 egg whites	4	0	0	
1 cup spinach, mushrooms, tomatoes (veggie omelet)	0	1	0	
Totals	4	1	0	
Dinner				
4 oz (112 g) chicken (dark)	4	0	0	
1/2 cup (57 g) green beans	0	1	0	
1 cup tomato and cucumber salad	0	1	0	
1 Tbsp (15 mL) Isabel's Famous Salad Dressing	0	0	1	
Totals	4	2	1	
Totals	17	6	3	

Day 10

Food	Protein	Carbs	Fat	Notes
Breakfast				
3 slices bacon (pork or turkey)	3	0	0	
1 slice sprouted whole grain bread	0	1	0	
1 tomato, sliced	0	1	0	
Totals	3	2	0	
Snack				
1/2 oz (14 g) brazil nuts (6-8)	1	0	0	
1/2 oz (14 g) macadamia nuts (6-8)	1	0	0	
Totals	2	0	0	
Lunch				
4 oz (112 g) scallops	4	0	0	
2 oz (57 g) avocado	0	0	2	
1 cup raw vegetables (spinach, cucumber, celery, peppers) made into a salad with lettuce	0	1	0	
2 tsp (10 mL) extra virgin olive oil and vinegar or lemon to dress the salad	0	0	2	
1 small green apple	0	1	0	
Totals	4	2	4	
Snack / Post Workout				
2 scoops BioTrust protein powder with water and ice	3	0	0	
1 banana	0	2	0	
Totals	3	2	0	
Dinner				
5 oz (112 g) ground turkey to use for turkey burger	5	0	0	
1 cup peppers and onions	0	1	0	
1 cup (90-180 g) sauteed spinach	0	1	0	
3 tsp (15 mL) coconut oil	0	0	0	
Totals	5	2	0	
Totals	17	8	4	

Day 11

Food	Protein	Carbs	Fat	Notes
Breakfast				
2 soft boiled eggs (or hard boiled)	2	0	0	
1 cup (100 g) steamed cauliflower	0	1	0	
2 oz (57 g) avocado	0	0	2	
Totals	2	1	2	
Snack				
2 Tbsp (28 g) nut butter	2	0	0	
1 cup baby carrots	0	1	0	
Totals	3	1	2	
Lunch				
4 oz (112 g) canned tuna (dark)	4	0	0	
1 cup celery, carrots, and red peppers	0	1	0	
1 Tbsp (15 mL) extra virgin olive oil	0	0	3	
1 cup (166 g) sliced strawberries	0	1	0	
Totals	4	2	3	
Snack / Post Workout				
4 oz (112 g) sliced turkey	4	0	0	
1 cup (90 g) cooked broccoli	0	1	0	
1 small green apple	0	1	0	
Totals	4	2	0	
Dinner				
4 oz (112 g) chicken (dark)	4	0	0	
1 cup (100 g) sauteed garlic broccoli	0	1	0	
1 cup raw vegetables (tomatoes, onions, carrots, celery) made into a salad with lettuce	0	1	0	
3 tsp (15 mL) extra virgin olive oil	0	0	3	
Totals	4	2	3	
Totals	16	8	8	

Day 12

Food	Protein	Carbs	Fat	Notes
Breakfast				
3 oz (84 g) leftover chicken (dark)	3	0	0	
1 cup (100 g) sauteed spinach	0	1	0	
2 tsp (10 mL) coconut oil - use for cooking spinach or eat raw	0	0	0	
1 small green apple	0	1	0	
Totals	3	2	0	
Snack				
1 oz pumpkin seeds	2	0	0	
Totals	2	0	0	
Lunch				
4 oz (112 g) ground buffalo (made into meatballs)	4	0	0	
Sauteed garlic tomatoes (1 whole tomato)	0	1	0	
1 cup (155 g) spaghetti squash	0	2	0	
2 tsp (10 mL) coconut oil - use for cooking tomato or eat raw	0	0	0	
Totals	4	3	0	
Snack / Post Workout				
2 scoops BioTrust Protein Powder	3	0	0	
1 cup (156 g) cooked rice cereal (hot cereal made from rice)	0	1	0	
Totals	3	1	0	
Dinner				
5 oz (142 g) tilapia	5	0	0	
2 oz (57 g) avocado	0	0	2	
1 cup (100 g) broccoli	0	1	0	
1 cup raw vegetables (cucumber, celery, green peppers) made into a salad with lettuce	0	1	0	
3 tsp (15 mL) extra virgin olive oil	0	0	3	
Totals	5	2	5	
Totals	18	8	5	

Day 13

Food	Protein	Carbs	Fat	Notes
Breakfast				
3 slices bacon (pork or turkey)	3	0	0	
1 egg	1	0	0	
1 tomato, sliced	0	1	0	
Totals	**4**	**1**	**0**	
Snack				
1 oz (28 g) raw walnuts (14 halves)	2	0	0	
Totals	**2**	**0**	**0**	
Lunch				
2 whole eggs + 2 egg whites + 1 Tbsp Dijon mustard + 1 tsp olive oil (to make egg salad)	4	0	1	
1 cup raw vegetables (cucumbers, celery, peppers, carrots) made into a salad with lettuce	0	1	0	
1 Tbsp Isabel's Famous Salad Dressing	0	0	1	
1/2 cup (76 g) green peas	0	1	0	
Totals	**4**	**2**	**2**	
Snack / Post Workout				
4 oz (112 g) sliced turkey breast	4	0	0	
Romaine lettuce leaves (make turkey, lettuce wraps)	0	0	0	
Dijon Mustard	0	0	0	
1 small green apple	0	1	0	
Totals	**3**	**1**	**0**	
Dinner				
5 oz (142 g) cooked chicken breast	5	0	0	
1 cup peppers and zucchini	0	1	0	
1 cup tomato and cucumber salad	0	1	0	
1-2 tsp (10-15 mL) wheat free soy sauce	0	0	0	
1 Tbsp Isabel's Famous Salad Dressing	0	0	1	
Totals	**5**	**2**	**1**	
Totals	**19**	**6**	**3**	

Day 14

Cheat Day

What can I eat on my cheat days?

You can eat whatever you like without gorging yourself. Don't eat until you are overly full at each meal. You can eat whatever foods you would until you are satisfied, just be reasonable. Two slices of pizza is a meal, but a whole pie is not! A slice of cake is a great dessert, not the whole cake! (I think you get the point).

What I do on my cheat days is just eat as I feel like it all day. I don't plan like I would on all my other days and I eat whatever I am craving. For example, I may wake up and make pancakes, have sushi for lunch followed by some cookies, and go out to dinner and choose whatever appeals to me on the menu (including dessert). As you can see, I do not eat with reckless abandon, but I don't plan my healthy meals like I do on the other days of the week.

The Shopping Guide

Getting Started

Shopping can sometimes be overwhelming. I get it. Since it is my goal to make this way of eating simple and easy, I have created this detailed shopping guide to help you navigate the supermarket and find your essential healthy food items in a quick and cost efficient way.

This guide was truly designed to make your transition to healthy food as effortless as possible.

My goal is not only to teach you how to shop for quality food, but to save you money at the same time (and who doesn't want to save money!) It will also save you an incredible amount of time while shopping.

Throughout this guide, I mention specific product brands. I have researched these brands and personally recommend them based on their effectiveness and their fit within the program. If you cannot find these brands in person or order them online, you can make substitutions using your judgment and principles you've learned here. However, I strongly recommend you use these brands, as I have already determined that these brands deliver on their promises.

Staple Foods Shopping List

The following is a list of food items you will use most frequently. You can take this list to the store to ensure you keep your house stocked with the basics. This list should be used as a starting point for your own shopping list, based on which foods you like to eat and which you prefer to avoid. Also, meal plans or individual recipes may call for additional or more specific items.

Produce
- **ORGANIC** - Read more about the importance of going organic, as well as which fruits and vegetables are most important to purchase organic here:
  http://www.beyonddiet.com/Members/Articles/6-Organic-Food

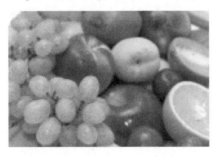 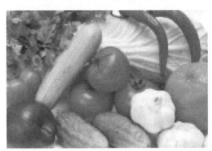

Meat/Poultry
- **Grass-fed, organic beef** purchase online here:
  http://go.beyonddiet.com/grasslandmeats
- **Organic Chicken**
- **Organic Turkey**

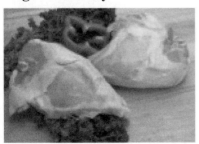 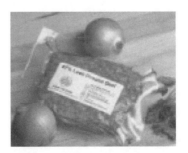

Seafood

- **Wild Fish** - purchased online here: http://go.beyonddiet.com/vitalchoice
- **Shrimp, Crab and Lobster**

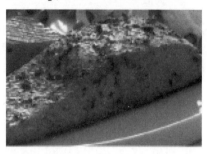 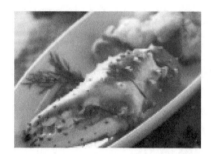

Dairy & Eggs

- **Organic Eggs**
- **Raw** (or Organic) **Milk**
- **Raw** (or Organic) **Butter**
- **Raw** (or Organic) **Cheese**
- **Organic Plain or Organic Greek Yogurt**

*For more information, refer to the Dairy chapter of the manual

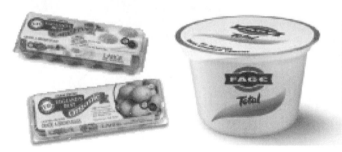 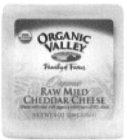

Grains
- **Ezekiel Sprouted Whole Grain (SWG) Bread**
- **Ezekiel Cereal**
- **Quinoa**
- **Rice**

*For more information, refer to the Grains chapter of the manual.

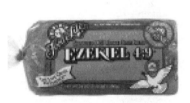 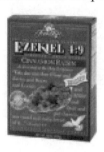 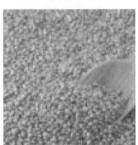

Nuts & Nut Butter
- **Raw Nuts**
- **Raw Nut Butters** - A nut butter is a spread made from crushed nuts (ex: raw almond butter)

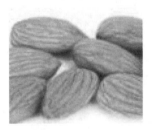 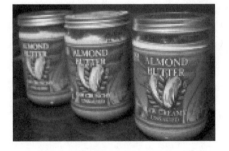

Oils (for dressings and cooking)

- **Extra Virgin, Unrefined Coconut Oil** purchase online here: http://go.beyonddiet.com/coconutoil
- **Extra Virgin Olive Oil (EVOO)** purchase online here: http://go.beyonddiet.com/orderoilolive

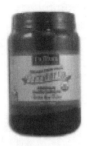 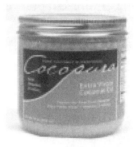 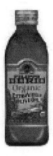

Sweeteners

- **Stevia**
- **Xylitol**

*For more information, refer to the Sweeteners chapter of the manual.

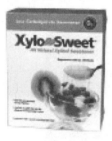

Flours

- **Almond Flour**
- **Coconut Flour**
- **Spelt Flour**

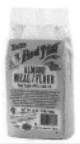 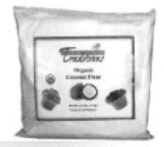 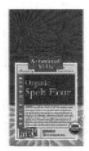

Beverages

- **Coconut Milk** find a recipe here:
  http://www.beyonddiet.com/Members/Recipes/Homemade-Coconut-Milk
- **Almond Milk** find a recipe here:
  http://www.beyonddiet.com/Members/Recipes/Homemade-Almond-Milk
- **Organic Tea:**
  - Rooibos Tea
  - Wu-Long Tea
- **Organic Coffee** purchase online here:
  http://www.beyonddiet.com/Members/Articles/Organic-Coffee

Condiments & Seasonings

- **Organic Condiments** (ketchup, mustard, etc.) **with no added sugar purchase online here:**
  http://www.beyonddiet.com/Members/Articles/Trinity-Hill-Farms-Sauces
- **Unrefined Sea Salt**
  - AztecSeaSalt™, purchase online here:
    go.beyonddiet.com/aztecseasalt
- Most **Herbs and Spices** used in cooking are fine to continue using.

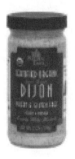
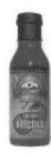
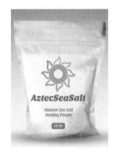

Supplements

- **Athletic Greens** purchase online here:
  www.beyonddiet.com/shop/Athletic-Greens-Super-Food
- Prograde Krill Oil purchase online here:
  www.beyonddiet.com/shop/Krill-Oil
- Protein Powders (optional)
  - BioTrust, purchase online here:
    www.beyonddiet.com/shop/Biotrust-Protein-Powder

*For more information, refer to the Supplements chapter of the manual

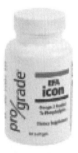
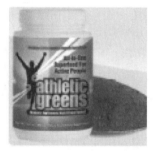
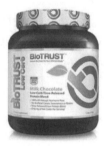

Understanding The Universal Layout

Whole Foods. Wegman's. Trader Joe's. Safeway. These supermarket chains may seem very different at first glance, but they all have one major similarity - their store layout. All grocery stores, no matter how big or small, follow a universal store structure. Think about the inside of your favorite, local supermarket. When you walk through the front door, you most likely walk into the produce section first. After the produce section, you will see the seafood section. Right next door is the meat department, where you'll find chicken, beef, lamb and pork. To the left of the meat department is where you'll find dairy and eggs. Usually to the left of the dairy section you'll find fresh baked breads.

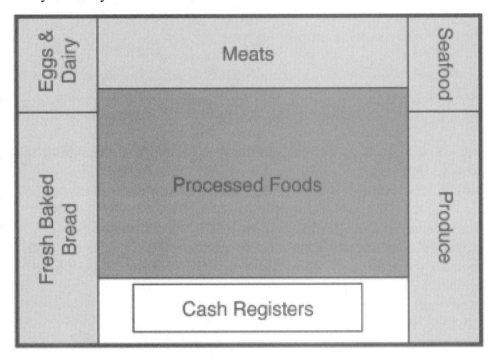

Pretty cool, huh? I bet you didn't realize that virtually all supermarkets purposely design their stores the same way.

This shopping guide follows this design as well, so that you can easily In order to make things as easy as possible for you while you're shopping, navigate through the store from the very first page. Understanding the design of a supermarket is key to learning how to shop properly. I will elaborate on this further in the next section.

The place you should spend 90% of your time

In the above section, I mentioned the universal supermarket design. All grocery stores have a universal layout, regardless of whether it's a health food store, an organic supermarket or your neighborhood grocery store.

I am specifically referring to the foods on the perimeter aisles. All perishable items (produce, meat, seafood, dairy and fresh baked breads) are located on the "perimeters," or the edges of the store.

The perimeters are where you should spend at least 90% of your time. Why? Perishable foods are unprocessed, whole foods and, therefore, have the most nutrients and minerals.

One of the keys to achieving success with Beyond Diet is consuming delicious foods in their whole food forms. Whole foods nutritionally sustain you so that you lose weight and stay healthy at the same time.

Ironically, it's the food with the shortest shelf life that costs the most money. However, this guide will show you that healthy food does not have to leave you with a hefty grocery bill.

Throughout this guide, I will teach you how to make wise decisions in the food aisle and how to stock a healthier kitchen. You'll have complete access to the most nutritionally-balanced, budget-conscious food choices available!

I've listed the best possible options in each category in order of ***best choice, second best, and good choice.***

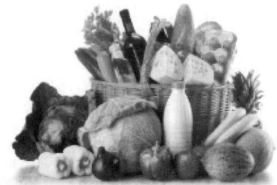

Your first lesson begins in the next section - produce.

The No-Nonsense Way to Selecting Quality Foods

Produce

Produce comes in every color of the rainbow, and it's as delicious as it is nutritious. The absolute **best choice** for produce is local produce. You may be surprised that my first choice wasn't organic produce. What most people do not realize is that many small local farms grow their produce without synthetic pesticides, but they cannot afford the USDA organic certification.

You may think that you can only purchase local produce at the farmer's market, but that's not true. Many supermarket chains proudly feature local produce. If you're not sure if your chain carries it, just ask.

- The advantages of local produce are:
- It's the freshest produce possible;
- You are helping to support your local economy and your local farmer;
- Buying local produce means you're eating "in season;"
- You are reducing the pollution in the environment.

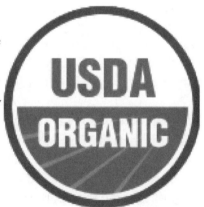

Organic is **second best** to non-synthetically pesticide grown local produce. Make sure you see the USDA Certified Organic or the USDA Organic green label (like the one to the right).

If money is no object, then by all means, purchase all of your produce in the organic section. However, if you want the **healthiest options available on a budget**, pay special attention to the last three paragraphs of this section.

Conventional produce is a ***good choice*** and last on the list in terms of most nutritious. Conventional produce does contain synthetic pesticides; however, not all conventional produce contain the same level of pesticides. You can save money and reduce your exposure to pesticides by purchasing fruits and vegetables lowest in pesticides. The link below lists the dirtiest and cleanest produce. The "dirty dozen" contain 12 types of produce with very high pesticide levels. It's important that you buy these fruits and vegetables organic. The "cleanest" produce lists 20 types of produce with the lowest levels of pesticides - you can buy this produce conventional.

You can view a list of produce with the highest and lowest pesticides levels online here »
http://www.beyonddiet.com/Members/Articles/6-Organic-Food

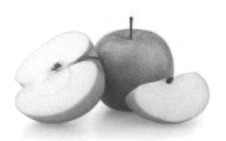

Seafood

Seafood, also known as the "protein of the sea," is delicious, versatile and loaded with healthy Omega 3 fatty acids. Selecting ideal fish and seafood is crucial for optimum health benefits.

Wild caught seafood is the only seafood that I recommend. Farm raised salmon are often loaded with high levels of polychlorinated biphenyl (PCB) and are artificially colored using canthaxanthin and synthetic astaxanthin (which is not fit for human consumption).

In addition to being wild caught, you should regularly consume seafood with low mercury levels, such as salmon, cod, and herring. Fish like tuna, swordfish, and shark, although delicious, have significantly higher mercury levels - you should only eat these on occasion. I have provided a list of fish and their corresponding mercury levels at the end of this section.

My recommendation rating in this section will be based on whether seafood is fresh, frozen, or canned.

The ***best choice*** for seafood is fresh, wild caught seafood. The fish should not have a fishy odor, and the flesh should be firm to the touch. The flesh should spring back easily if you press on it. Make sure the sign on the fish explicitly says "wild caught." Ask the person behind the seafood counter to press on the flesh so you can judge the quality for yourself. If you are buying shellfish, such as shrimp, crabs, clams, mussels, octopus or squid, make sure that these are wild caught as well. If you are not sure if they are wild caught, always ***ask*** the employee behind the counter.

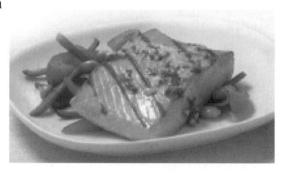

The ***second best*** choice for seafood is frozen seafood. Frozen seafood, in most cases, is just as healthy as fresh seafood because it is usually frozen within hours after it is caught. As with the wild seafood, make sure it clearly says "wild caught" on the packaging. Another added perk of frozen seafood is that it's ***usually less expensive*** than fresh seafood. Trader Joe's, in particular, is an affordable choice for a great variety of frozen seafood.

A ***good*** choice and even more cost efficient choice for seafood is wild caught canned seafood. Oysters, wild-caught salmon, clams, low-mercury tuna, and sardines are packed with flavor, protein and Omega 3's. Canned seafood is significantly cheaper than both fresh and frozen seafood, allowing you to indulge even if you are on a strict budget. When you buy canned seafood, there are two things to look for: make sure that the seafood comes in BPA-free cans and that it is packed in pure olive oil or water. BPA (bisphenol A) is a chemical present in the lining of the can, and has been known to interfere with hormones.

Two trusted brands for delicious and safe canned seafood are Vital Choice and Crown Prince.

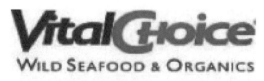

VitalChoice

WILD SEAFOOD & ORGANICS

Savor The Essence Of Purity

Purchase Vital Choice Online here: http://go.beyonddiet.com/vitalchoice
You can access a great chart for mercury levels here »
http://go.beyonddiet.com/vitalchoice

Meats

When you're in the meat aisle, read the labels of the meat very carefully.
The *best* choice for meats fits the below criteria:

- It's Organic
- It's Free-range
- It's Grass fed (pastured)
- It's Antibiotic free
- It's Hormone free

Why antibiotic and hormone free? Animals are routinely given growth
hormones to make them bigger, so they produce more meat (more meat
means more money). Feedlot cattle are kept in pens where they are living
on top of each other. In these types of unsanitary conditions, cattle often
become sick; in order to combat this, cattle are given antibiotics.

Make sure that you see *all* of these words on the label (please keep in
mind that grass fed primarily applies to meat, not poultry, such as chicken
or turkey). The meat should be fresh and should have a healthy color and
hue.

Grass fed meats are usually more expensive when you purchase them in
supermarkets, but cost significantly less when you purchase them directly
from the farm (I will elaborate more on this in a later section).

An added benefit of grass fed meats is that they contain higher amounts
of Vitamin E, Omega 3's, and a powerful fat buring compound, CLA
(conjugated linoleic acid) than conventional store-bought beef. A study
published in the American Journal of Clinical Nutrition proved that CLA
reduces body fat without compromising muscle. ***CLA found in foods,***

such as grass fed meats and grass fed raw dairy products, is far superior to any supplement on the market.

Grass fed meat is also heart-healthy (as you can see below).

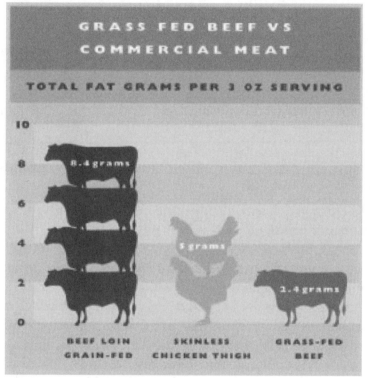

The second best choices for meats are those that are ***organic, free-range, and free of antibiotics and hormones.***

A ***good*** choice for meats, and the least expensive option for grocery bought meats, are those that are:

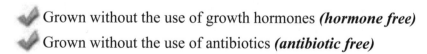

Grown without the use of growth hormones *(hormone free)*
Grown without the use of antibiotics *(antibiotic free)*

If you see the word "natural," don't be fooled. Natural does not represent livestock that have been raised without the use of hormones and antibiotics.

If you buy meats, such as bacon or cold cuts, always make sure that you purchase these items nitrate free.

US Wellness is an amazing and convenient resource for nutritious, mouth-watering organic and grass fed meats with zero hormones, antibiotics, and nitrates - delivered right to your door! Browse through prime cuts of chicken, beef, pork, lamb and even buffalo.

Purchase US Wellness products online here:
http://go.beyonddiet.com/grasslandmeats

Dairy/Eggs

Dairy - it's creamy, rich and yummy. And more importantly, the right dairy can be *very healthy* for you as well.

The *best* choice for dairy is raw, grass-fed dairy. Raw dairy (unpasteurized and unhomogenized) contains more Vitamins A, D, C and B vitamins than the pasteurized, homogenized store-bought version. Raw whole milk dairy also contains high levels of CLA and Omega 3 in its butterfat; in other words, this fat helps to dissolve *your fat*. The butterfat is also what gives the dairy a rich golden color and contributes to its rich, luscious and delicious taste! Many local farmers sell clean, nutritious, grass fed dairy (yogurt, cheese, cream, kefir, etc). If you are interested in purchasing raw dairy or would like to read about the facts behind raw dairy, pasteurization and homogenization, please visit http://realmilk.com.

The *second best* choice is store-bought pastured dairy that is antibiotic and hormone free (ideally unhomogenized). Brands like Organic Valley are available in many stores, and many of its dairy products (milk, cheese, heavy cream, butter) are grass fed (pastured).

A *good* choice for dairy is organic, antibiotic and BGH free (bovine growth hormone) that is not ultra-homogenized. Horizon is an organic brand that is sold nationwide in supermarkets.

For grass fed, healthy and scrumptious dairy delivered to your door, please visit US Wellness Meats online at: http://go.beyonddiet.com/grasslandmeats

Eggs

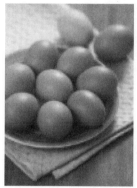

The criteria for buying eggs are very similar to those for buying meats. The **best** choice for eggs are grass fed (pastured), free range eggs, preferably from a local farm. These eggs are taken from chickens allowed to freely graze on grass and bugs (which is part of their natural diet), without being kept in cages. Not only do the eggs taste better, but the chickens are treated humanely and the eggs contain higher vitamin amounts than their store bought counterparts. You can see this in the deep rich yellow orange color of the yolk.

The **second best** choice is organic eggs rich in Omega 3s (ideally free-range or cage free). These chickens are fed organic feed that has higher Omega 3 levels than standard eggs.

A **good** choice for eggs are organic eggs (ideally free-range or cage free). These eggs come from free-range or cage free chickens (chickens who spend some time outside of a cage) that are fed natural feed.

Breads

When choosing breads, fresh with the least preservatives is always best. However, here at Beyond Diet, I want your foods to sustain your taste buds and your health. For this reason, I recommend breads that use organic sprouted grains. Why sprouted? Sprouting begins the enzymatic action that starts to break down the gluten, which makes the wheat more easily digestible and better tolerated by people with gluten sensitivities. Gluten, a protein found in wheat and grains like barley and rye, can cause digestive upsets for many people. As a matter of fact, according to a

February 2003 study from the Archives of Internal Medicine, over 1.5 million Americans have celiac disease, a digestive condition aggravated by gluten.

When selecting breads, you must read the labels carefully. Look for grains in their most natural form, preferably sprouted. For example, wheat should ideally read as *"sprouted wheat"* on the ingredients list. If you see ingredients such as "refined wheat flour" or "unbleached enriched wheat flour," look elsewhere because these last two ingredients are forms of processed wheat.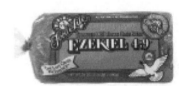

The *best* choice for bread is one made from sprouted grains. A great and tasty example of sprouted whole grain (SWG) bread is Food for Life's Ezekiel 4:9 organic bread. The list of ingredients reads as follows: Organic Sprouted Wheat, Organic Sprouted Barley, Organic Sprouted Millet, Malted Barley, Organic Sprouted Lentils, Organic Sprouted Soybeans, Organic Spelt, Filtered Water, Fresh Yeast, Sea Salt.

Notice how the ingredients are simple, easy to read and understand. You should also notice how the grains listed are in their most natural form. Looking for more variety at the breakfast table than a slice of toast? Ezekiel Bread is versatile and comes in multiple varieties and flavors to fit your meal plan, such as Cinnamon Raisin Bread, English Muffins, Rolls, and Tortillas.

This bread can be found in most health food stores and supermarkets (often located in the freezer section). If your health food store or supermarket does not carry this brand, you can find it here: http://go.beyonddiet.com/bread »

It's not necessary for you to buy this specific brand, but I highly recommend it. The important thing for you to do is to closely read the ingredients of any bread that you buy.

Rice Bread

If you're unable to obtain sprouted grain bread, your *second best* choice would be rice bread, made from rice flour. These breads are gluten and wheat free and easily digestible by the body. The first ingredient for this type of bread should be "Brown Rice Flour." If you can't find rice bread with brown rice flour on the label; rice flour is your next best option.

Spelt Bread

A *good* choice, if you are not extremely intolerant to wheat or gluten, is spelt bread (spelt belongs to the wheat family and does contain gluten but is sometimes much easier to digest for people who have a difficult time digesting wheat).

You want to ensure that the first ingredient is "spelt flour."

Make sure to carefully read the label of your bread to ensure that it does NOT contain these ingredients:

- ✗ Hydrogenated Oil
- ✗ High Fructose Corn Syrup
- ✗ Bleached, enriched flour
- ✗ Wheat Gluten
- ✗ Artificial Flavor
- ✗ Sugars or Artificial Sweeteners (Aspartame or Sucralose).

Healthy Condiments -
Add on the Flavor, Not the Additives

Who doesn't like condiments? They're versatile, full of flavor and they enhance our food. While some condiments taste good, they're not necessarily good for you. This section of my guide explores condiments that elevate your taste buds and your health.

Salts

Quality salt is essential for taste and for health. Contrary to popular belief, salt is actually GOOD for you, but, not just any salt will do. Table salt and most sea salts have been processed and contain many chemical additives. These salts are stripped of their healing benefits and are not beneficial to your health.

Healthy salts are **_unrefined_** and untouched. It's important that you only purchase salt that states that it is unrefined. You can easily identify unrefined sea salt because of its unique color; natural sea salt comes in all colors ranging from grey to black. One example is AztecSeaSalt™. This salt is a light grey color because it's unprocessed. It's dried naturally by the sun and the wind. The lack of processing ensures that the trace minerals are intact. This salt supplies more than 80 trace minerals needed for optimum biological health and cell function.

AztecSeaSalt™ is a trusted brand that I highly recommend. This salt is not sold in stores, but you can purchase it here: go.beyonddiet.com/aztecseasalt

Make sure your salt does NOT contain any of the following:

- ✗ Sugar (added to stabilize Iodine and as anti-caking chemical)
- ✗ Aluminum silicate.

Sweeteners

To see how these sweeteners compare to each other, view the chart at the end of this section.

Moderation is the key to life, and when it comes to sugar, this statement is even more true. When you eat sugar, you should do so in moderation. If you do eat foods with sugar, the best choices for natural sugars are unprocessed sweeteners like raw honey, brown rice syrup, coconut sugar and pure maple syrup (Grade B). Remember, natural sugars are still sugar. Don't be fooled into thinking that because it sounds healthy, you can eat as much of it as you want. An even better alternative to natural sugars is a sugar free, healthy, natural plant based substitute called stevia.

Brown Rice Syrup

Brown rice syrup is the sweet golden syrup by-product of cooking brown rice in water, and then evaporating most of the water. It's also gluten and wheat-free.

Raw Honey

Honey, in its raw and unrefined form, contains a host of phytonutrients and enzymes that have a multitude of beneficial attributes. Refining honey uses heat, which destroys all of these enzymes and nutrients. Honey does not cause the rapid blood sugar rise and fall that white sugar does.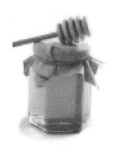

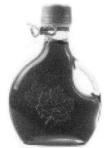

Pure Maple Syrup (Grade B)

Pure maple syrup is a natural sugar made from the sap of maple trees. There are two grades of pure maple syrup: Grade A and Grade B. Grade B maple syrup has a more pronounced maple flavor than Grade A. It also has a thicker consistency than grade A. Because of its rich flavor, you need less of this syrup, so you'll consume less overall sugar compared to Grade A syrup. Use both grades in moderation.

Coconut Sugar

Coconut sugar is a sugar made from the coconut flower. It is boiled down and is available in three forms: sugar blocks, soft paste, or in granular form.

Stevia

Many stevia formulations are available (e.g., liquid, powder, and powder plus inulin fiber). The liquid extract is ideal for cold beverages; the powders are ideal for baking and hot liquids. Read the packages to determine which product is right for you and the correct amounts to use in recipes. Sources include local health food stores and online.

Make sure your stevia product does NOT contain maltodextrin, dextrose, or any sugar derivative. Some stevia powders include inulin fiber. This is OK, as it's a natural fiber also found in fruits and vegetables (although some people complain that this particular fiber gives them gas and bloating). Make sure you monitor your own body's response.

Xylitol

Some people like the taste of stevia; for others, it's an acquired taste. If you don't enjoy the taste of stevia, you may want to try xylitol instead. Again, always be sure to monitor your body's response to any new food, as some people do not digest xylitol well.

The ingredients label should only list "xylitol" and no other additives.

Below is a comparison chart of the above sweeteners. All sweeteners have a Glycemic Index (GI). A GI rating measures how you blood sugar levels will react to certain foods. The higher the number, the more drastic your blood sugar spike will be.
* In liquid form

**In powder form

Oils and Fats

I recommend that you buy virgin cold-pressed, unrefined oils only (mainly olive and coconut). You should avoid all other vegetable oils (canola, soybean, etc) - the average human diet contains way too much of these ingredients. For more in-depth information about this subject, please reference the Fats chapter in the Beyond Diet manual.

Sweeteners Comparison Chart	Raw Honey	Brown Rice Syrup	Coconut Palm Sugar	Pure Maple Syrup (Grade B)	Stevia (Sugar Free)	Xylitol (Sugar Free)
Glycemic Index (GI) Rating	30	25	35	54	0	7
Available in powder and liquid form					✓	✓
Is minimally processed	✓	✓	✓	✓	✓	✓
Number of calories per serving (per teaspoon)	20	23	15	17	0	10
Contains trace minerals	✓	✓	✓	✓	✓	✓
Ideal for Cold Beverages			✓		✓ *	✓
Ideal for Baking and Hot Beverages	✓	✓	✓	✓	✓ **	✓

Extra Virgin Olive Oil

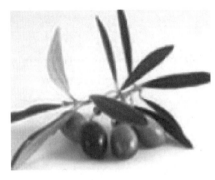

Olive oil is flavorful oil that is derived from - you guessed it - olives. Organic olive oil is naturally pressed and has superior taste.

For medium-heat cooking (sautéing) and use straight from the bottle (on salads and cooked foods), choose organic extra-virgin olive oil. It should be cold-pressed, cloudy (unrefined), and sold in a dark bottle.
Sources include local health food stores and the following:

Vital Choice, purchase online here:
http://go.beyonddiet.com/vitalchoice

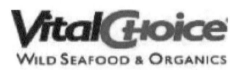

WILD SEAFOOD & ORGANICS

Savor The Essence Of Purity

Virgin Coconut Oil

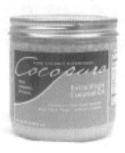

Coconut oil has a thermogenic effect on the body, which means that it helps you to burn fat. It's also a great energy booster!

The healthy saturated fats in coconut oil have anti-microbial properties that help keep gut flora (good bacteria) in check. Coconut oil also contains high amounts of lauric acid which helps to keep your immune system strong against certain viruses, like the flu. When used topically the fatty acids in the oil deeply penetrate and moisturize your skin. A University of Kerala study reveals that virgin coconut oil speeds up your skin's collagen turnover rate. Collagen is a protein that holds the skin together, repairs broken skin, and keeps your skin wrinkle-free (added benefit, ladies). The high collagen turnover rate coconut oil provides helps to accelerate healing for burns and cuts, while the antibacterial properties of lauric acid provide a barrier against infection and germs.
Tip: For kitchen burns and cuts, always keep a small jar of virgin coconut oil near the sink.

You will receive the most benefit from coconut oil that smells and tastes of fresh coconuts.

This type of oil *should* be:

 Organic

Virgin

Cold-pressed

This type of oil *should not* contain any chemicals (including hexane).

My personal recommendations for *coconut oil* are:

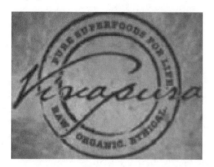 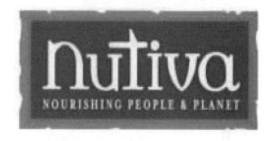

Get CocoPura online at: http://go.beyonddiet.com/ordercoconutoil
Get Nutiva online at: http://go.beyonddiet.com/coconutoil

Grass Fed Butter

You should also use butter for cooking, in recipes or on top of vegetables. For high heat cooking, I recommend butter and virgin coconut oil.

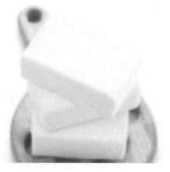

Organic raw butter made from grass fed cows would be your best choice. If you are unable to find raw, organic grass fed butter, organic butter from grass fed cows is your second best choice. If either is not available, organic butter can also be used.

Make sure the ingredients on the label are:

- Organic Cream (or milk)
- Salt (I purchase unsalted and then add my own Sea Salt)

Grass fed butter contains vitamin K2, which is important for healthy teeth, bones and may reduce heart disease and certain cancers.

Nut Butters

Choose nut butters (e.g., almond, walnut, cashew, or macadamia nut) made from raw (not roasted) organic nuts.
Sources include local health food stores and the following:

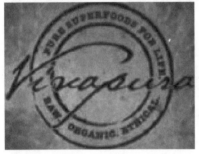

Get VivaPura online at: http://go.beyonddiet.com/shopvivapura

If you are unable to find these brands, make sure that you choose a brand with a minimal amount of ingredients.

For example, an ideal Almond Butter ingredient label should read:

Raw (Organic) Almonds.

And that's it!

Some nut butters add salt, but it is best to find those without added salt. Stay away from brands that list the first ingredient as:

Dry Roasted Almonds

Natural Peanut Butter is a bit more difficult to obtain in its raw state. I encourage you to try some of the other nut butter varieties (walnut, cashew, macadamia nut) or make your own Homemade Peanut Butter made from raw peanuts. Below is a simple, delicious recipe.

Homemade Peanut Butter

1 cup raw peanuts
4 Tbsp water
1-2 Tbsp of raw honey depending on taste (2 Tbsp is very sweet)
1 1/2 Tbsp coconut or extra virgin olive oil

Put all ingredients into your food processor and blend. It will become spreadable but not creamy.

Processed Foods

As a general rule, you should eat as little processed food as possible.

The main rule is to look at the product's ingredients in addition to the nutritional content in the serving column. The nutrition label can show that a product has 0g of trans-fat per serving even though it is made with partially hydrogenated oils (listed in the ingredients). Make sure you read *each item* under the ingredients.

Avoid items with hydrogenated or partially hydrogenated oils (anything hydrogenated or partially hydrogenated is trans fat), high fructose corn syrup, artificial preservatives and flavors, artificial sweeteners (Equal, Splenda, Sweet and Low, etc.), MSG, high sodium contents and high sugar content (more than 15g per serving).

When you do eat processed food, stay clear of/limit consumption of foods with the following words in the ingredients. ***These are hidden names for MSG.***

MSG	Gelatin	Calcium Caseinate
Monosodium Glutamate	Hydrolized Vegetable Protein	Textured Protein
Monopotassium Glutamate	Hydrolized Plant Protein	Yeast Extract
Glutamate	Autolyzed Plant Protein	Yeast Food or Nutrient
Glutamic Acid	Sodium Caseinate	Autolyzed Yeast

Likewise, eliminate/reduce your consumption of processed foods containing the below ingredients. ***The below are hidden names for sugar.*** Many processed and boxed foods contain more than one of these ingredients in one product.

Dextrose	Sorbitol	Maltose
High-Fructose Corn Syrup	Corn Syrup	Invert Sugar
Malic Acid	Sucrose	Carob Powder
Maltodextrin	Glucose Syrup	Rice Malt
Diglycerides	Concentrated Fruit Juice	Levulose

Healthy Snacks -
Sabatoge-Free Satisfaction

This section covers healthy snacks - yes, there is such a thing. I only recommend snacks that work with you in your weight loss efforts - not against you. These snacks are as convenient as they are tasty.

Jerky - No Slim Jims Allowed

Jerky is one of the most versatile and convenient ways to get a great source of protein. I'm not talking about the Slim Jims you buy in 7-11. Natural jerkies are available without nitrates or additives. They 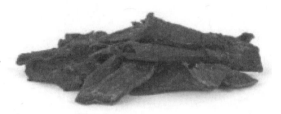 even come in an array of flavors, such as beef, buffalo, turkey and even wild salmon! The protein keeps you nice and full until your next meal. I recommend natural jerky from US Wellness.

Get Natural Jerky online here:
http://go.beyonddiet.com/glbuyjerky

Greek Yogurt (Full Fat) - Fat is Your Friend

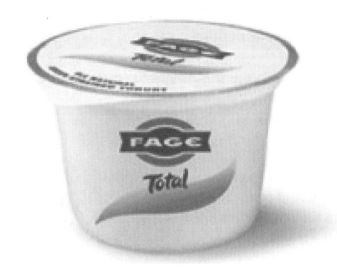

Yogurt is a commonly eaten fermented food. Fermented foods are a necessity in our diet. They help keep a balance of healthy bacteria or flora (probiotics) within your gut.

Full Fat Greek yogurt tastes so delicious, you may forget that it's good for you. Greek yogurt has a thick, custard-like consistency that has more protein than plain yogurt. The full fat in the yogurt keeps you fuller for longer between meals. Fage is a brand available nationwide. I recommend Fage Total, which is the full fat version of the yogurt. For a guilt-free touch of sweetness, add stevia or a tablespoon of raw honey and a handful of raw nuts for an added protein boost.

For those who prefer the taste of traditional yogurt, your best choice would be raw, grass fed yogurt. Your second best choice for healthy yogurt is organic, grass fed yogurt. If you are unable to locate one of the first two choices, a good choice is an organic, hormone and antibiotic free store bought brand, such as Stonyfield. Opt for the plain flavor, as this has the least amount of sugar (you can always add your own fruit and/or natural sweetener/sugar substitute at home).

Smoked Oysters and Sardines

Get your protein and Omega 3s in one place. Naturally smoked oysters and sardines, by Crown Prince, provide a whopping 10 grams of protein per can! Both products are packed in extra virgin olive oil for a good source of heart healthy monounsaturated fats.

Raw Nuts

Raw nuts, such as almonds, walnuts and cashews are an excellent source of protein.

Get Raw Nuts here:
http://go.beyonddiet.com/tfmrawnuts

Raw Cheese

Raw milk cheese is a great source of CLA, a fat-fighting compound that occurs naturally in this food. It is also a good source of protein. Pair this treat with a low sugar fruit, like an apple, for a mid-afternoon delight.

Get Raw Cheese here:
http://go.beyonddiet.com/glbuyrawcheese

Beverages

Although water is an ideal beverage, let's face it - every now and then you want something different. There are more and more healthy beverages being released on the market each day. Below is a brand that I recommend.

Honest Teas
Honest Teas is a NY based beverage company that was launched in 1998. Its product line is centered on organic teas and juice blends. Honest Teas recently launched a no calorie line that flavors its drinks with stevia. So far they have two flavors: Classic lemonade and passion fruit green tea.

Organic on the Cheap: 20 Ways to Save Big Bucks on Organic Groceries

Quality costs more - it's not a theory, it's a fact. This applies to food as well. These days, everyone can benefit from saving money. Fortunately for you, there are numerous ways to significantly save money at the grocery register, and I've listed the top 20 resources. For added convenience, most of these resources are available within your own community (if you live in a city, you can also access many of these resources).

I care about all of my clients and I want to do everything in my power to ensure your success on your weight loss program. One of the easiest ways that I can do this is to help save you money so that you can lose weight and become healthier, without unloading your wallet.

1. Warehouse Shopping Costs

Warehouse discount clubs have long been appreciated by the public for saving money on bulk items like paper towels and toilet tissue. Now you can add organic items to that list. Costco and BJ's are just two examples of warehouse stores that carry organic foods, such as meats, produce, dairy and eggs, soups and smoothies.

Chances are you probably already have a membership to one of these clubs. If you don't, you can get twice the value for half the price by splitting the membership with a friend or family member. Another option is to go shopping with someone who does. When you've finished shopping, give the person with the membership the money for your portion of the groceries!

If you live in a part of the country with a Super Walmart, be sure to check out their organic food and produce sections as well.

2. Farmer's Markets - Farmer Knows Best

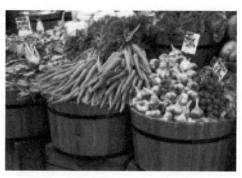

Farmer's markets are a great resource within most communities. The produce is local, the farmers are friendly, and the quality is outstanding. Many farmers don't us synthetic pesticides for their crops. Since crops are grown locally, they don't have to be transported far distances, which means that your food won't lose valuable nutrients during shipping. Best of all, if you have a question about a particular item, you can always ask the source directly!

Because produce is local, farmer's market prices are generally cheaper than organic and even conventional produce.

3. Community Supported Agriculture (CSA) - Produce Delivered to Your Door

CSAs are a new way to bring the farm to your door, literally. CSAs allow you to pay for a membership to purchase a share from a local farm for a season. Every week you'll receive a box of seasonal produce (the CSA will give you a list of the seasonal produce beforehand so you know how much of each item you'll be receiving). Prices for the membership (over the course of the season) are usually much lower than purchasing these items at a supermarket.

CSAs also offer other food items such as meats, dairy and homemade bread.

Not only is this option convenient, it's also cost effective. If you are a single person, you can save even more money by spitting the membership (and groceries) with another friend. To find a local CSA in your community, please visit: www.localharvest.org/csa

4. Go Directly to the Farm

Going directly to the farm allows you to purchase the freshest cuts of meats available - directly from the source. It's also the best place to get the cheapest price per pound. When supermarkets buy meats, they pay for shipping, packaging and the equipment to cool the meat. The store then passes these costs onto you, the consumer. Buying the meat directly from the farmer allows you to bypass the middle man, the grocery store, so that you can save money. This translates to less money per pound for your meat.

Many local farms feed their livestock grass and their chickens natural feed, so your food will still be nutritionally dense - for much less! If you want to confirm what the animals are eating, you can ask the farmer these questions directly.

Ask your family, friends and people in your neighborhood if they would like to split up the meat of a cow, pig, chicken, or lamb. Let them know that they will most likely pay less per pound than going to the store - I'm sure you'll have no problem finding at least 10 willing participants. Many of these farms give you the option to buy dairy directly from them as well.

To find the closest farm to you, please visit:
eatwild.com »

5. Build Your Own Chicken Coop

As I've previously stated, pastured eggs are superior to conventional eggs in both nutrition and taste. If you live in the country you can make sure that you always have access to the freshest eggs around. How is this possible? By building your own chicken coop. You don't have to be an engineer to build a chicken coop; there are many do-it-yourself ebooks that can show you how to build your own chicken coop, step by step. For a great source visit: go.beyonddiet.com/chickencoop

6. Buy in Bulk Online

Buying meats in bulk is not something you only have to do at the farm; you can also buy bulk quality meats online. Buying online allows you to split the costs of the food with your friends and neighbors, and have the meat delivered directly to you. This is a great option if you're busy and don't have time to drive to your nearest farm.

I recommend US Wellness for bulk quality meats:
http://go.beyonddiet.com/grasslandmeats

7. Eat Fewer Processed Foods

This may seem like an obvious solution, but you'd be surprised at how much money you shell out on snacks and boxed foods. Cutting out processed foods is one of the easiest ways to save money on your grocery bill. You can test this option yourself. For one month, buy 1/2 to a 1/4 of the processed foods that you'd normally buy. At the end of the month, compare your previous month's bills with your bills for that month - I guarantee you'll see a difference.

8. Make More Delicious Meals at Home; Eat Out Less

Another easy way to save money is to make more of your meals at home. This includes lunches. On Sunday, set aside a few hours to cook your food for the week. Make about 6-8 simple meals, wrap them well and freeze them. Multiple meals allows you to rotate your meals, so you don't have to keep eating the same foods over and over again. Reward yourself by going out to dinner at your favorite restaurant at the end of the month, and bank the remainder of the money that you've saved.

9. Whole Nutrition = The Sum of All of The Parts

Use all of the parts of the animal, including the organs. Not only are these parts nutritionally dense, but they're cheap! Make sure that the organs are from pastured (grass fed) animals.
http://go.beyonddiet.com/grasslandmeats

10. Is There a Butcher in the House?

Find a good quality butcher in your neighborhood for cheap bones and organs. Many people no longer make their own stocks, and many people do not eat organ meats (offal). Butchers will most likely throw these items away. They'll probably sell these items to you for very little money; if you're lucky, they may even give them to you for free! Remember to request grass fed bones and offal as they're the best choice.

11. Grow Your Own Veggies

One of the best ways to save money on produce is to grow your own at home. Growing your own garden is easier than you think; many people have been doing this as a hobby for years. Ebooks make tending your own garden easier than ever before.

I highly recommend "Food for Wealth" - If you are new to the world of organic gardening, this book breaks down the art of growing your own produce into simple steps. Once you've mastered the basics, I recommend a second book "Aquaponics4you." This book seriously improves your organic gardening techniques to yield more vegetables for your efforts. The combination will give you a one, two punch to getting the best value for your home grown organic garden.
Food4Wealth: www.food4wealth.com
Aquaponics4You: www.aquaponics4you.com

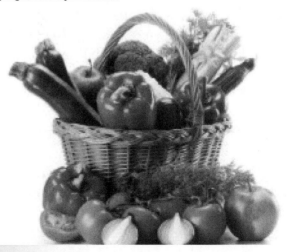

12. Co-ops

A food co-op is a collectively owned grocery store. A food co-op is a great central location for natural and organic foods more affordable for co-op members. Many co-op memberships require you to work at the store for a few hours a month in exchange for a free membership! Co-op members often receive discounts on many items within the store.

To find a natural co-op near you, please visit http://www.coopdirectory.org

13. Private Label Brands

Look for sensibly priced Private Label Brands (PLB) at your supermarket. 365 Everyday is Whole Foods' PLB. The ingredients in most of their items are outstanding - in fact, all Whole Foods PLB items are natural, and most are organic! And the price can be a much as $3-4 less than their brand label counterpart!

14. Bone up on Marrow Bones

Marrow bones are inexpensive, luscious and super nutritious. They contain over 40% of monounsaturated fats (the same fats in olive oil and avocados). Many high class restaurants are now serving this treat as an expensive, decadent appetizer, but you can indulge for much less. Ask your local butcher, or the farmer if you are buying your meat directly from the farm to throw in some marrow bones with your order. Below is a recipe for roasted bone marrow:

Roasted Bone Marrow with Garlic

8-12 grass fed beef bones with marrow (3 to 4 pounds total)
1 cup fresh parsley, roughly chopped
1 head of garlic
2 shallots, thinly sliced
2 teaspoons capers
1 1/2 tablespoons extra virgin olive oil
2 teaspoons fresh lemon juice
Celtic Sea Salt
Sprouted Whole Grain bread, toasted

Preheat the oven to 375 degrees. Cut the top off the head of garlic and place in the middle of a sheet of aluminum foil. Drizzle with a couple teaspoons of olive oil and add a pinch of salt. Close the foil around the garlic, creating a tight pouch, and place the garlic into the oven for 45 minutes. Remove from the oven. Open the pouch and allow to cool for a couple of minutes. When the head of garlic is cool enough to the touch, squeeze out the warm, soft garlic and spread onto the toast with the marrow.

Preheat the oven to 450 degrees. Place bones, cut side up, onto a foil-lined baking sheet or in an ovenproof cast iron skillet. Cook until the marrow is soft and has begun to separate from the bone - about 15 minutes. (Stop before the marrow begins to drizzle out). Meanwhile, combine parsley, shallots and capers into a small bowl. Just before the bones are ready, whisk together the olive oil and lemon juice and drizzle the dressing over the parsley mixture until the leaves are coated.

Place the roasted bones, parsley salad, salt and toast onto a large plate. To serve, scoop out the marrow, spread onto the toast, sprinkle with a tiny bit of salt and top with the parsley salad.

15. Dairy You Can Make at Home

If you are an avid cook or feel particularly adventurous in the kitchen, you can really stretch your dollars and make your own grass-fed yogurt and butter from pastured or raw milk.

For a DIY quality butter recipe, please refer to this link:
http://www.foodrenegade.com/how-to-make-butter

Yogurt recipe provided by: http://nourishedkitchen.com/raw-milk-yogurt

16. Bake Your Own Bread

You can also make your own delicious, sprouted bread at home. For more money saving goodness, use this simple, yet hearty recipe.

Gluten Free Rice Bread Recipe

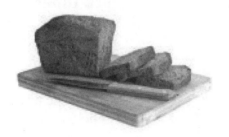

1 cup brown rice
7/8 cup water
1 egg
1 teaspoon baking powder
1/4 teaspoon

Soak the rice in the water overnight (6-12 hours). Grind the rice and water mixture in a blender until the rice particles in the batter reach the consistency of fine salt. Add egg, baking powder and salt to the batter, mix well.

Bake COVERED for 30 minutes in a well-oiled eight-inch iron skillet or a casserole dish (a well-seasoned cast iron skillet can't be beat for baking with rice).

17. Freeze It

Buy fruits and vegetables in bulk when they're in season. Double wrap the produce in freezer resistant wrapping, and place them in freezer bags to keep out freezer burn and lock in the flavor.

18. Bartering food with neighbors and friends

Save money on groceries by trading food items with your friends and neighbors in your community. This is also great if you have more food items than you or your family needs.

19. Online Coupons

You don't have to go searching your Sunday paper to clip coupons - unless you want to. There are great online resources like http://www.organicfoodcoupons.com and http://www.ecobunga.com, which provide many ways to save money on organic foods.

20. Have a Potluck Dinner!

This is the easiest and most social way to save money. Once a week (or however often you choose), have a healthy potluck dinner with your family, friends and neighbors using organic foods. Assign one or two dishes to each person. For the price of two side dishes, you'll have access to a full banquet of delicious, nutritious food!

Recipes

Recipes

This guide includes some of my favorite recipes, adapted from cookbooks and online sources. Because Beyond Diet is not a diet in the traditional sense but a new way of eating that you want to adopt for life, it is essential that you keep your meals tasty, interesting, and creative. Eating the same foods again and again leads to boredom and abandonment. To prevent this from happening, I highly encourage you to try at least one new recipe per week that suits your meal plan. Also, be adventurous and try some foods that you have never tried before.

With all of the recipes presented here (and with any other recipe you may choose to use), adhere to all the principles taught in the manual. For example, organic ingredients are always best. Whenever possible, choose free-range, hormone- and antibiotic-free, fresh, and wild meats, poultry, eggs, and fish. Don't fear salt, but do use an unrefined sea salt or, preferably, Celtic sea salt. Oils should be cold expeller-pressed. Water should be pure and filtered. And the only breads you should consumer should be made from organic sprouted whole grains (e.g., Food for Life brand's Ezekiel 4:9 products).

Also, remember that allowable food servings and portion sizes differ for each person, depending on metabolic type and the number of calories required daily. Please adjust recipe portions to suit your meal plan, as instructed in the Chapter on Daily Meal Planning, according to the Allowable Servings Guide and the Food Choices charts. For example, if you are a Carb Type allowed four 1-oz servings of protein for dinner and a chicken recipe makes 6-oz servings (or doesn't specify a portion size), eat only 4 oz of chicken with your meal.

Remember, fresh food is best, and the more whole and natural the food you eat, the healthier you will be—and the better you will feel. Bon appétit!

Table of Contents

Recipes

Beverages

Tea Juice

Drink this when you have a sugar craving. It's a great substitute for unhealthy diet sodas and other sweet beverages.

Ingredients

5-6 bags Caffeine-Free Herbal Tea (e.g., peach, mint, chamomile, or fruit tea)

3 quarts (2.84 liters) Boiling Water

To taste Stevia Powder (or liquid)

Directions

Pour water over tea bags in a large pot. Add stevia while tea is hot. (Adjust amount according to the desired sweetness.)

Let the tea cool, remove tea bags, transfer tea to a serving pitcher or individual water bottles, and refrigerate.

Dressings, Marinades, Seasonings, & Sauces

Basic Salad Dressing

Sally Fallon, Nourishing Traditions

Makes: ~ 3/4 cup (180mL)

Ingredients

1 tsp (5mL) Dijon-style mustard, smooth or grainy

2 Tbsp (30mL) + 1 tsp (5mL) wine vinegar

½ cup (120mL) olive oil

1 Tbsp (15mL) flax seed oil

Directions

Whisk mustard into vinegar. Add olive oil in a thin stream, whisking constantly until oil is emulsified. Whisk in flax oil, and use immediately.

Variation: Mix 1 tsp (5mL) of finely chopped fresh herbs (e.g., parsley, tarragon, thyme, basil, or oregano) into the basic recipe after the mix has emulsified.

Lemon Pepper Dressing

Used in the Summer Salad recipe

Makes: ~ 3/4 cup (180mL)

Ingredients

2 Tbsp (30mL) fresh lemon juice

1 Tbsp (15mL) wine vinegar

1 clove garlic, minced

½ (120mL) cup olive oil

1 Tbsp (15mL) flax seed oil

1 dash stevia powder

¼ (1.25mL) tsp salt

½ tsp (2.5mL) cracked black peppercorns

Directions

Place all ingredients in a bowl, and whisk vigorously until the mixture emulsifies.

Use-It-On-Everything Marinade

This delicious marinade works equally well on veggies, fish, poultry, and beef. It's particularly tasty on London broil, tri-tips, or chuck steak.

Prep Time: 15 min
Marinating Time: overnight
Makes: enough for 20 lb of food

Ingredients

1 red onion, sliced

1 whole head garlic, cloves minced

1 cup (240mL) lemon juice

1¼ cups (300mL) red wine vinegar

4 cups (950mL) olive oil

4 tsp (40mL) salt

4 tsp (40mL) ground white pepper

4 tsp (40mL) freshly ground black pepper

4 tsp (40mL) paprika

3 tsp (30mL) dried basil

4 tsp (40mL) Worcestershire sauce

Directions

Mix all ingredients until well blended. Pour over food, and marinate overnight.

Tip: Place food in a gallon-size plastic zipper-top bag, cover with marinade, and seal. This package travels well in coolers and is less cumbersome than a pan in the refrigerator. Flip the bag several times while marinating to cover the food evenly.

Cilantro Marinade

This marinade is delicious on Grilled Swordfish or eggplant.

Makes: ~ 1/2 cup (120mL)

Directions

Mix all ingredients together.

Ingredients

1 bunch cilantro, leaves only, finely chopped

Juice of 1 lemon

½ cup (120mL) olive oil

¼ tsp (1.25mL) freshly ground black pepper

3 cloves garlic, minced

Caribbean Jerk Rub

Dry rubs are low-calorie, low-carbohydrate seasonings that are simple yet flavorful. Use this recipe on Grilled Caribbean Chicken.

Ingredients

6 Tbsp (60g) minced garlic (or garlic powder)

6 Tbsp (60g) minced onion

6 Tbsp (50g) dried minced onion (or onion powder)

2 Tbsp (30mL) allspice

2 Tbsp (30mL) dried thyme

2 Tbsp (30mL) ground cinnamon

2 tsp (10mL) ground nutmeg

2 Tbsp (30mL) Hungarian paprika

1 packet Sweet Leaf stevia powder

1½ tsp (7.5mL) ground habanero pepper

1 Tbsp (15mL) dried ground chipotle (or ground red chili pepper)

Zest of 2 lemons

Directions

Mix together all ingredients. Store in covered container, refrigerated, up to 1 month.

Béarnaise Sauce

Properly made, béarnaise sauce never attains more than medium heat, so the enzymes in the egg yolks are preserved. So delicious with meats and grilled fish, this sauce is worth mastering—and it's not difficult. Used in the Grilled Swordfish recipe.

Makes: 1¼ cup (295mL)

Ingredients

5 egg yolks, at room temperature

2 Tbsp (12g) finely chopped shallots (or green onions)

4 oz (1 stick) butter, cut into pieces

2 Tbsp (30mL) white wine vinegar

2 Tbsp (30mL) dry white wine (or vermouth)

1 Tbsp (15mL) finely chopped fresh tarragon (or 1 tsp (5mL) dried tarragon)

fresh lemon juice to taste

pinch of salt

pinch of freshly ground black pepper

Directions

In a small saucepan, combine the shallots, tarragon, vinegar, and wine. Bring mixture to a boil, and reduce to ~1 Tbsp of liquid. Strain into a bowl and set aside.

In a small bowl, whisk the egg yolks and set aside.

Set the bowl with the reduced liquid over a pan of hot water over low heat. Piece by piece, add about half the butter to the liquid, whisking constantly until melted. Add the egg yolks slowly, drop by drop or in a thin stream, whisking constantly. Add the remaining butter, and whisk until well amalgamated. Sauce should be warm and slightly thickened. Remove from heat and whisk in lemon juice, salt, and pepper.

Set the bowl set over hot water to keep sauce warm, whisking occasionally, until ready to serve.

Vegetable Dishes

Summer Salad

This salad is best made several hours before serving. The secret to its success is to cut the vegetables in a fine dice. A food processor makes that task quick and easy.

Servings: 6

Ingredients

3 tomatoes

2 cucumbers, peeled, quartered lengthwise, and finely chopped

2 bunches green onions, finely chopped

2 green peppers, seeded and finely chopped

1 bunch celery, finely chopped

1 bunch radishes, finely chopped

1 Tbsp (30mL) finely chopped fresh parsley (or chives)

¾ cup (180mL) Lemon Pepper Dressing

Directions

Place the dressing in a large bowl. Add celery, cucumbers, green onions, peppers, and radishes. Toss well with dressing, cover, and refrigerate several hours.

Just before serving, slice the tomatoes thinly, then cut the slices in half. Arrange slices around the outer edge of six plates, and mound some salad in the center of each. Sprinkle with chopped parsley.

Garlicky Steamed Stuffed Artichokes

This dish is messy to eat but delicious.

Servings: 4

Ingredients

4 artichokes

4 cloves garlic, minced

2 cups (120g) breadcrumbs (make your own from fresh or stale sprouted whole grain bread)

½ cup (120mL) olive oil (or melted butter)

salt and freshly ground black pepper to taste

Directions

Remove the artichoke stems and place, stem side down, in a vegetable steamer or a large pot containing about 1 inch (2.5cm) of water. Steam, covered, no more than 30 minutes, or until just barely tender. Place artichokes in a colander to drain, stem side up.

Mix olive oil with garlic, breadcrumbs, salt, and pepper. Pull artichoke leaves open a bit, and snip points off leaves with kitchen shears. Press stuffing between leaves. Return to steamer for another 5–10 minutes.

Asparagus with Sesame Seeds

Servings: 6

Ingredients

2½ lb (900g) asparagus, trimmed

2 Tbsp (30mL) sesame seeds, lightly toasted

2 Tbsp (30mL) minced shallots

2 Tbsp (30mL) olive oil (or melted butter)

1 lemon

salt to taste

Directions

Preheat oven to 400°F (204C).

Place oil and asparagus in an ovenproof baking dish, and toss asparagus to completely coat with oil. Bake for about 8 minutes, shaking the dish every 2 minutes or so. Add the shallots and sesame seeds, shake the dish again, and bake 1 minute more.

Transfer asparagus to heated serving bowl, and squeeze lemon juice all over. Season to taste with salt.

Vegetable Dishes

Vegetable Frittata

A frittata is like a no-flip omelet or a no-crust quiche—a fast egg dish that can be made with any combination of vegetable, meat, and cheese that you can imagine.

Prep Time: 15 min
Servings: 4

Ingredients

8 medium eggs

4 cups (600g) chopped low-GI vegetables (e.g., broccoli, cauliflower, zucchini, artichoke hearts, asparagus, spinach)

3 tsp dry mustard (or 2 tsp (10mL) prepared mustard)

2 Tbsp (30mL) minced fresh marjoram

2 Tbsp (30mL) butter (or coconut oil)

¾ cup (110g) chopped red onion

1 lb (450g) mushrooms (or red peppers), sliced

1 tsp (5mL) freshly ground black pepper

1 tsp (5mL) Spike vegetable seasoning (or salt)

¼ (60mL) cup milk

Directions

Heat butter in large skillet over medium-high heat. Add onion and mushrooms and cook, stirring, for 1–2 minutes, or until onions are translucent.

Add chopped vegetables and marjoram. Sauté until vegetables turn bright green and begin to soften. Reduce heat to medium or medium-low.

Meanwhile, break eggs into a small bowl. Add milk, mustard, and black pepper. Use a fork to break yolks gently, without whisking (mixture will look marbleized), and pour eggs over vegetables in skillet. Cook over medium heat until eggs are set.

Basic Spaghetti Squash

Spaghetti squash is tasty low-carbohydrate substitute for pasta.

Ingredients

1 spaghetti squash (any size)

butter, to taste

salt and freshly ground black pepper, to taste

Directions

Preheat oven to 350°F (177C).

Cut spaghetti squash in half lengthwise; remove and discard seeds. Place squash, cut sides down, in a baking pan with about ½ inch (13mm) of water. Bake for about 1 hour, or until tender when pricked with a fork.

Let squash cool slightly, then remove the strands of flesh, bit by bit, with a fork. Mix in butter, salt, and pepper.

Variation: Serve topped with grated Parmesan cheese, pesto, or tomato sauce.

Vegetable Dishes

Butternut Squash Puree with Pecans

Servings: 6

Ingredients

3 medium butternut squash

3 eggs, lightly beaten

2 Tbsp (30mL) butter, melted

1–2 Tbsp (15-30mL) butter (to grease the dish)

¾ cup (110g) raw pecans, chopped

¼ tsp (1.25mL) nutmeg

salt to taste

Directions

Preheat oven to 350°F (177C).

Cut squash in half; remove and discard seeds. Place squash, cut side down, in a buttered ovenproof baking dish with about ½ inch of water. Bake about 1 hour, until tender when pricked with a fork.

After squash is cooked, scoop out flesh into a food processor and blend until smooth. Add eggs and nutmeg, and season to taste with salt. Transfer puree to an ovenproof serving dish. Pour the melted butter over the puree and sprinkle on pecans. Bake for about 30 minutes.

Wilted Spinach

Servings: 3

Ingredients

1 bunch (~10 oz) (280g) whole fresh spinach leaves

butter, to taste

Directions

Cut off the stems on the spinach and wash well in water—even if prewashed, so that the leaves are moist. Place in a large pot, cover, and heat over a medium heat. (Do not add more water to the pot; the water on the leaves will be sufficient to steam the spinach.)

When spinach begins to simmer, reduce heat to low. Cook several minutes, until leaves are just wilted.

Using a slotted spoon, transfer spinach to a heated serving bowl. Press spinach with the back of the spoon and discard any liquid. Make a few cuts through the spinach, and top with a generous pat of butter.

Vegetable Dishes

Butternut Squash Puree with Pecans

This delicious and elegant accompaniment to beef may be prepared in advance.

Servings: 8

Ingredients

8 large whole fresh white button mushrooms

1 cup (150g) steamed spinach

2 Tbsp (20mL) butter

2 Tbsp (30mL) olive oil

1 bunch green onions, finely chopped

1–2 Tbsp (15-30mL) butter (to grease the dish)

¼ tsp (1.25mL) nutmeg

salt and freshly ground black pepper to taste

Directions

Preheat oven to 350°F (177C).

Chop cooked spinach, place in a strainer, and press out liquid.

Wash mushrooms. Remove and finely chop stems; set aside whole mushroom caps.

Sauté mushroom stems with green onions in butter and olive oil until tender. Add the spinach, and cook another minute or so, mixing well, until all moisture has evaporated. Add nutmeg, and season to taste with salt and pepper.

Fill the hollow of each mushroom cap with a spoonful of stuffing, and place in a buttered ovenproof baking dish. Add ¼ inch (6mm) of water to the dish, and bake for about 20 minutes.

Seasoned Wilted Spinach

Servings: 6

Ingredients

2 bunches fresh spinach

1 clove garlic, minced

1 Tbsp (15mL) pine nuts

1 Tbsp (15mL) butter

1 Tbsp (15mL) sun-dried tomato flakes (optional)

Directions

Steam spinach as described for Wilted Spinach. Melt butter with garlic, pine nuts, and tomato flakes. Pour over spinach, mix slightly, and serve.

Vegetable Dishes

Baked Sweet Potatoes

Servings: 4

Ingredients

4 whole (4-ounce) (113g) sweet potatoes

4 tsp (20mL) butter

salt to taste

Directions

Preheat oven to 350°F (177C).

Prick each sweet potato in several places with a fork. Bake for 1½ hours, or until soft when pricked with a fork.

Mash the flesh with butter and salt.

Sweet Potato Dollars

Servings: 4

Ingredients

3–4 whole (4-ounce) (113g) sweet potatoes

2 Tbsp (30mL) olive oil

1 Tbsp (15mL) melted butter

salt to taste

Directions

Preheat oven to 350°F (177C).

Peel potatoes, and slice crosswise into ¼-inch rounds.

Combine butter and olive oil, and brush two cookie sheets with half of this mixture. Arrange the rounds in one layer, then brush tops with the remaining butter–oil mixture. Season lightly with salt. Bake about 45 minutes.

Vegetable Dishes

Sautéed Zucchini

Like all members of the squash family, zucchini is ruined by boiling. Even steaming gives watery results. Instead, sauté slices in butter or olive oil and finish with a squeeze of lemon and salt and pepper.

Servings: 4

Ingredients

6 medium zucchini, washed and trimmed

2 tsp (10mL) salt

2 Tbsp butter (30mL) (or olive oil)

juice of ½ lemon

salt and freshly ground black pepper to taste

Directions

Slice zucchini into thin matchstick-like pieces (or use the small julienne disk of a food processor). Add salt, stir well to mix, and let stand 1 hour.

Rinse zucchini with water in a colander, and squeeze dry in a tea towel.

Melt butter slowly in a heavy skillet over low heat. Raise heat to medium, and sauté zucchini for about 1 minute. Remove to a serving dish, and season with lemon juice, salt, and pepper.

Zucchini with Tomatoes

Servings: 4

Ingredients

2 medium zucchini, washed and trimmed

2 Tbsp (30mL) butter, divided

2 Tbsp (30mL) olive oil, divided

2 medium onions, peeled and chopped

2 medium tomatoes, peeled, seeded, and chopped

1 or 2 cloves garlic, minced

¾ tsp (3.75mL) salt

½ tsp (2.5mL) dried thyme

½ tsp (2.5mL) freshly ground black pepper

Directions

Cut zucchini into quarters lengthwise, then slice each section into thin quarter-rounds. Mix with salt, and let stand about 1 hour. Rinse zucchini in a colander, and pat dry.

Warm 1 tbsp butter and 1 tbsp olive oil in a large skillet, and sauté zucchini in batches over medium-high heat until golden. Remove and set aside zucchini.

Sauté onion in 1 tbsp butter and 1 tbsp olive oil over medium heat until tender. Add tomatoes, raise heat, and cook a few minutes until liquid is almost all absorbed. Add cooked zucchini, garlic, thyme, and pepper. Sauté about 1 minute more to mix flavors. Don't overcook zucchini!

Roasted Red Pepper Dip

Prep Time: 5-10 min
Cook Time: 30 min
Makes: 2 cups

Ingredients

1 cup (220g) home made mayonnaise (link to recipe)

1 cup (150g) roasted red peppers

12 oz (340g) artichoke hearts (unmarinated)

1/8 tsp (.125mL) garlic powder

1/3 cup (30g) raw parmesan cheese, grated

2 Tbsp (30mL) red onion

Directions

Preheat oven to 350F (177C).

Place everything in the food processor and process until smooth.

Transfer to the baking dish and bake for 30 minutes. Serve warm.

Baba Ganouj - Roasted Eggplant Dip

A classic Middle Eastern dip made of roasted eggplant. Delicious!

Servings: 4

Ingredients

4 Tbsp (60mL) tahini

4 Tbsp (60mL) plain yogurt (optional)

2 lbs (900g) eggplant

2 cloves garlic, minced

1 Tbsp (15mL) olive oil

½ cup (120mL) fresh lemon juice

Directions

Slice the eggplant in half lengthwise, score the face of each half with the knife, and brush each face with olive oil.

Bake or grill: If baking, place eggplant face up on cookie sheet and put on oven pre-heated to 450F (232C). If grilling, place eggplant face down over medium heat.

Cook for 40-50 minutes, until eggplant is black and soft. (Smaller eggplants will take less time.) Lay out on the platter to cool.

With a spoon, remove the eggplant flesh from the skin and place in blender or food processor. Discard skin.

Blend/process on low speed for a few seconds, until consistent.

Mix in remaining ingredients, taste, and add more tahini, lemon juice, and/or salt as necessary. Chill for about an hour.

Arrange baba ganouj in a shallow bowl, drizzle with olive oil and sprinkle with parsley. Serve with vegetables or sprouted grain toast.

The broiling/grilling step is the key to delicious baba ganouj: it makes the eggplant taste rich and smoky.

Baba ganouj keeps pretty well in the fridge, except for one thing: the garlic gets stronger with each passing day. If you're not planning to eat the baba ganouj right away, you might want to cut down on the amount of garlic for this recipe.

Pumpkin Soup

This spicy pumpkin soup is a good way to use up all of that pumpkin left over from Halloween.

Cook Time: 30 min
Servings: 6

Ingredients

2 potatoes, peeled and diced

2 Tbsp (30mL) olive oil

1½ pounds (675g) pumpkin (weighed before trimming)

1 leek, washed, trimmed, and sliced into rings

1 qt (1L) vegetable stock

½ tsp (2.5mL) salt

1 tsp (5mL) pepper

½ - 1 tsp (2.5-5mL) cayenne pepper

Directions

Cut the top off the pumpkin, scoop out the seeds and strings, peel the shell, and dice the flesh.

Sauté the pumpkin, leek, and potatoes in olive oil for 5 minutes, stirring frequently.

Add vegetable stock and bring to a boil. Cover and boil the soup for 15 minutes, until potatoes are soft.

Purée the soup and add spices and lemon juice. Ladle into bowls and serve.

You can use leftover jack-o'-lanterns, but the soup will taste noticeably better if made with smaller, more flavorful pumpkins.

Poultry

Basic Roast Chicken

This recipe is quick, easy, and delicious! Refrigerate or freeze leftover chicken for quick meals during the week.

Prep Time: 10 min
Servings: 6

Ingredients

1 6- to 8-lb (2700-3600g) roasting chicken

1 Tbsp (15mL) butter, softened

1 medium garlic clove, minced

2 tsp (10mL) minced fresh thyme leaves

4–5 grinds black pepper

¾ tsp (3.75mL) salt

Directions

Note: For a golden breast, turn the chicken before the last 30 minutes of cooking.

Preheat oven to 350°F (177C).

Wash chicken, and remove fat from inside cavity.

In a small bowl, combine butter, garlic, salt, pepper, and thyme to make a paste; rub it over the chicken. Place chicken in roasting pan, breast side down.

Roast, uncovered, basting frequently, for approximately 1½ hours (about 20 minutes per pound). Chicken is done when leg pulls off easily and juices no longer run red when chicken is pricked with a fork. Remove chicken from pan and let rest, covered, for 5–10 minutes.

Cut chicken into serving pieces, or slice and serve with gravy on the side. Remove skin before eating.

Tip: Deglaze the roasting pan and make gravy, if desired, thickened with 1½ tbsp arrowroot dissolved in 2 cups (475mL) water.

Steamed Chicken and Vegetables

Steaming the chicken with vegetables is a simple, healthy method that reduces excess fat, cooking time, and kitchen mess.

Prep Time: 15 min
Servings: 4

Ingredients

6 scallions (or green onions), cut into thirds

1 1-inch (2.5cm) piece fresh ginger root, peeled, sliced, and cut into matchsticks

1 medium garlic clove, minced

1 medium head savoy cabbage, shredded

3–4 grinds black pepper

2 large boneless chicken breast halves, cut in half

2 tsp (10mL) coconut oil (or butter)

½ cup (120mL) chicken stock

¾ cup (110g) baby carrots, split lengthwise

½ cup (120mL) coarsely chopped curly (or flat-leaf) parsley

1 tsp (5mL) salt (or Spike vegetable seasoning, or Herbamare seasoned salt)

Directions

Note: The author suggests cooking in a Bundt pan as the steamer; however, a bamboo steamer tray or a metal colander also can be used in a covered stockpot.

Bring 2–3 inches (5-7.6cm) of water to a boil in a large stockpot. Lower heat to simmer.

Place shredded cabbage in the bottom of a Bundt pan. Meanwhile, combine carrots, ginger, garlic, scallions, parsley, and chicken in a large bowl. Add oil, and season with salt and pepper. Toss to mix. Pile mixture evenly on top of cabbage.

Place Bundt pan into simmering water. Pour chicken stock over the chicken and vegetables, cover, and steam lightly for 18–20 minutes.

Grilled Caribbean Chicken

Prep Time: 10 min
Servings: 5

Ingredients

2 broiler-fryer chicken halves

1 Tbsp (15mL) coconut oil (or butter)

6 Tbsp (90mL) Caribbean Jerk Rub (page 11)

Directions

Preheat grill to medium.

Rub broiler-fryer halves lightly with oil and then with Caribbean Jerk Rub.

Cook chicken, turning every 15–20 minutes until tender, approximately 1–1½ hours.

Bare Bones Low-Fat Chicken Salad

(David Kirsch, *The Ultimate New York Body Plan*)

Prep Time: 15 min
Servings: 4

Ingredients

4 oz (113g) poached chicken breast, cut into 1-inch cubes

2 tsp (10mL) Dijon-style mustard

2 Tbsp (30mL) chicken stock

1 tsp (5mL) finely chopped parsley

1 Tbsp (15mL) sliced almonds, coarsely chopped

¼ cup (60mL) coarsely chopped celery

1 or 2 dashes hot pepper sauce

salt and freshly ground black pepper to taste

Directions

In a medium bowl, mix chicken, celery, parsley, and almonds.

In another bowl, whisk mustard, stock, and hot pepper sauce together until well blended.

Combine mixtures, and stir well. Season with salt and black pepper.

Easy Grilled Chicken Breasts

Serve alongside grilled asparagus or a side salad.

Prep Time: 10 min
Marinate Time: 1 hour
Cook Time: 15 min
Servings: 4

Ingredients

4 boneless skinless chicken breast halves

1 tsp (5mL) salt

1 tsp (5mL) freshly ground black pepper

¼ (60mL) cup olive oil

juice of 1 lemon

Directions

Rinse chicken thoroughly with cool water. Whisk olive oil, lemon juice, salt, and pepper in large bowl. Refrigerate chicken in marinade for 1 hour.

Preheat grill until it reaches medium heat.

Cook chicken for 6–8 minutes per side, or until golden brown.

Garlic- and Herb-Marinated Chicken Breasts

Marinate Time: 2 hours or overnight
Cook Time: 15 min
Servings: 4

Ingredients

6 boneless skinless chicken breast halves

5 cloves garlic, minced

1 Tbsp (15mL) olive oil

1 tsp (5mL) dried basil

1 tsp (5mL) dried thyme

1 tsp (5mL) dried oregano

1 tsp (5mL) dried tarragon

1 tsp (5mL) salt

1 tsp (5mL) freshly ground black pepper

juice and zest of 1 lemon

½ cup (120mL) olive oil

Directions

Mix the garlic, herbs, salt, pepper, lemon juice and zest, and olive oil in a large (1-gallon) plastic zipper-top bag. Add chicken, and marinate for at least 2 hours (up to overnight) in refrigerator.

Preheat a grill to medium-high.

Brush grate with oil. Sear chicken 5 minutes per side, or until its internal temperature reaches 165°F (74C).

Tomato-Fennel Chicken with Cauliflower and Olives

Prep Time: ~ 45 min
Servings: 4

Ingredients

8 boneless skinless chicken thighs

8 cloves garlic, thinly sliced2 tsp (10mL) olive oil

4 cups (600g) cauliflower florets

1 cup (240mL) dry white wine, divided

1 cup (240mL) chicken broth

1 cup (150g) pitted kalamata olives

28 oz (784g) crushed tomatoes (canned is fine)

1 Tbsp (15mL) chopped fresh parsley

1 tsp (5mL) fennel seeds

1 tsp (5mL) sun-dried tomatoes, minced

¼ tsp (1.25mL) salt

⅛ tsp (.125g) pepper

¼ tsp (1.25mL) ground cayenne pepper

zest of 1 lemon

Directions

Heat olive oil in a large pot over high heat. Brown chicken on both sides, cooking for about 3–4 minutes per side. Remove chicken from pot; reduce heat to low. Pour off excess oil.

To the same pot, add garlic and 1 Tbsp wine. Cook 1 minute. Stir in remaining wine, crushed tomatoes, broth, fennel seeds, cayenne, sun-dried tomatoes, zest, olives, salt, and pepper. Return chicken to pot. Increase heat to high to bring sauce to a boil. Reduce heat to low; cover pot. Simmer 25 minutes.

Stir in cauliflower florets. Simmer 10 minutes more, until chicken is cooked through and cauliflower is tender.

Remove chicken to a serving platter, and top with sauce. Sprinkle with fresh parsley.

Chicken Margarita

Servings: 4

Ingredients

1 tsp (5mL) ground cumin

1 Tbsp (15mL) chili powder

3 Tbsp (45mL) olive oil, divided

3½ lb (1575g) chicken pieces

½ cup (120mL) tequila, white or gold

½ cup (120mL) water

fresh cilantro leaves (for garnish)

juice of 3 limes

10 cloves garlic, finely chopped

Directions

In a large bowl, combine cumin, chili powder, lime juice, garlic, and 1 tsp olive oil. Marinate chicken pieces in this marinade for 20 minutes.

In heavy skillet, heat remaining olive oil. Brown chicken pieces on all sides. Add marinade, tequila, and water. Cook for approximately 10 minutes. Transfer chicken pieces to a platter.

Reduce sauce over high heat until it thickens to a good coating consistency, pour over chicken, and serve garnished with cilantro.

Chicken in Coconut-Lime Sauce

Servings: 4

Ingredients

4 bone-in chicken thighs

4 bone-in chicken drumsticks

3 Tbsp (45mL) coconut oil

2 dried red hot peppers

1 Tbsp (30mL) minced garlic

1 tsp (10mL) curry powder

½ cup (75g) sliced green onions

½ cup (75g) prepared salsa

½ tsp (2.5mL) salt

¼ tsp (1.25mL) freshly ground black pepper

13½ oz (395mL) (1 can) coconut milk

½ cup (120mL) fresh lime juice

½ cup (75g) grated coconut (for garnish)

a few lime slices (for garnish)

a few fresh red hot peppers (for garnish)

Directions

In large frying pan, warm coconut oil over medium-high heat. Brown chicken in batches, about 5 minutes on each side; remove from frying pan and keep warm.

To frying pan, add green onions, salsa, garlic, dried hot peppers, curry powder, salt, and black pepper; cook about 2 minutes, stirring, until onion is browned. Return chicken to pan; pour coconut milk and lime juice over chicken. Simmer over low heat about 30 minutes, or until fork can be inserted into chicken with ease. Remove and discard hot peppers.

Remove chicken to a platter. Garnish with lime slices and fresh red hot peppers, and sprinkle lightly with grated coconut before serving.

Coriander Chicken

Because cilantro is the leaf and coriander the seed of the same plant, either seasoning can be used in this recipe.

Servings: 4

Ingredients

1 small (3- to 4-lb) chicken, cut into pieces

1 Tbsp (15mL) butter

1 tsp (5mL) turmeric (or saffron)

1 sprig of fresh cilantro, finely chopped (or 2 tsp (1g) ground coriander)

1 cup (240mL) (or more) water

4 Tbsp (60mL) olive oil

4 large cloves of garlic, crushed

¼ lb (113g) purple olives, pitted

1 lemon, sliced

salt and freshly ground black pepper to taste

Directions

Brown the chicken in butter and oil in a large heavy skillet over medium heat. Add garlic, turmeric, salt, pepper, and cilantro. Cook about 10 minutes, turning chicken occasionally to distribute sauce evenly. Stir in enough water to cover (about 1 cup (240mL), and simmer over low heat until the chicken is tender, adding more water if necessary.

Add olives and lemon slices, and cook 8–10 more minutes, or until sauce is reduced.

Country Chicken

Servings: 4

Ingredients

6 tomatoes (canned with juice is fine)

4 slices bacon

2 cloves garlic, minced

1 small (3-lb) chicken, cut into 8 pieces

2 Tbsp (30mL) curry powder

1 green bell pepper, seeded and chopped

1 onion, chopped

1 cup (240mL) orange juice

¾ cup (110g) minced celery

½ tsp (2.5mL) dried thyme

½ (75g) cup raisins

½ cup (75g) almonds, toasted and chopped coarsely

¼ cup (40g) minced parsley

Directions

In a skillet, sauté the bacon until crisp, then drain on paper towels. With the hot bacon fat that remains in the pan, brown the chicken pieces quickly, a few at a time, turning often. Set the browned pieces aside.

Drain all but 2 Tbsp (30mL) of fat from the pan. Add the pepper, onion, garlic, and celery, and sauté for 5 minutes. Coarsely chop the tomatoes, and add to the pan with a little of their juice and the orange juice. Season with curry powder and thyme. Bring mixture to a boil, then reduce the heat and simmer for 5 minutes.

Return the chicken to the pan, and stir to cover them with sauce. Cover and simmer 30 minutes more.

Remove chicken to a platter. Spoon sauce over chicken, and garnish with raisins, almonds, and parsley before serving.

Poultry

Roasted Chicken with Rosemary & Garlic

Servings: 8

Ingredients

1 large (5- to 6-lb) roasting chicken

1½ Tbsp (22.5mL) minced garlic

1½ Tbsp (22.5mL) chopped fresh rosemary

1 Tbsp (15mL) olive oil

2 whole heads garlic

4 medium onions

Preheat oven to 450°F (232C)

Directions

Rinse chicken and pat dry. Remove and discard neck, giblets, and any excess fat. Loosen skin from breast and drumsticks. Place minced garlic and rosemary beneath skin. Lift wing tips up and over back; tuck behind chicken. Place chicken, breast side up, in a broiler pan.

Cut thin slices from the ends of each onion, and peel. Cut tops off garlic, leaving root end intact. Brush onions and garlic heads with olive oil; place around chicken.

Bake for 30 minutes. Reduce heat to 350°F (177C), and bake an additional 1 hour and 15 minutes, or until the internal temperature registers 180°F (82C).

Country Chicken

Servings: 4

Ingredients

2 Cornish game hens, split lengthwise

2 Tbsp (30mL) olive oil

2 Tbsp (30mL) butter, melted

2 cups (475mL) chicken stock

2 cups (300g) red (or green) seedless grapes

2 Tbsp (30mL) arrowroot mixed with 2 tbsp (30mL) water

½ cup (120mL) dry white wine (or vermouth)

salt and freshly ground black pepper to taste

Directions

Note: Arrowroot is a fine white powder that resembles cornstarch. Because it thickens when heated in liquid, it is an excellent ingredient in sauces.

Preheat oven to 375°F (191C).

Place game hens, skin side up, in a roasting pan. Brush with a mixture of butter and oil, and season with salt and pepper. Bake for about 1½ hours. Remove to a heated platter, and keep warm in the oven.

Pour wine into the roasting pan and bring mixture to a boil, scraping up any accumulated juices in the pan. Add chicken stock, bring to a rapid boil, skim, and let the sauce reduce for about 10 minutes. Add the grapes, and simmer about 5 minutes more. Add arrowroot mixture by the spoonful until the desired thickness is obtained.

Transfer game hens to individual plates, and pour sauce over to serve.

Poultry

Quick Turkey Cutlets

This tasty recipe could get dinner on the table in a hurry any weeknight.

Prep Time: 10 min
Servings: 4

Ingredients

4 tsp (20mL) butter (or coconut oil)

4 tsp (20mL) minced fresh rosemary (or 2 tsp crushed dried rosemary)

4–5 grinds black pepper

2 Tbsp (30mL) green olives, pitted, sliced in half

1¼ lb (560g) boneless turkey thighs

1¼ tsp (6.25mL) salt

¼ cup (60mL) lemon juice

Directions

Pound turkey (between pieces of waxed paper or plastic wrap) with large flat knife or meat mallet to an even thickness of ⅛ inch (3mm). Season with salt and pepper.

Melt butter in a large sauté pan or skillet over medium-high heat. Sear turkey cutlets on one side. Turn cutlets, and cook for 1 minute.

Season cutlets with rosemary, lemon juice, and olives. Cook for 2–3 minutes more. Remove cutlets to a serving platter and keep warm.

Scrape up any browned bits from the bottom of pan, and continue heating until sauce is reduced to about 2 Tbsp (30mL). Pour sauce over cutlets, and serve immediately.

Tarragon Turkey Burgers

These burgers are delicious! And not much more trouble than making beef burgers.

Prep Time: 5 min
Servings: 4

Ingredients

1 lb (450g) ground turkey

1 Tbsp (15mL) fresh (or dried) tarragon leaves

2 large eggs

2 tsp (10mL) Dijon-style mustard

½ tsp (2.5mL) Spike vegetable seasoning (or salt)

½ cup (75g) coarsely shredded zucchini

¼ cup (40g) chopped red onion

3 grinds black pepper

Directions

Preheat broiler or grill.

In a large bowl, combine all ingredients and shape mixture into patties.

Cook 5 minutes per side, or until browned. (Do not overcook.)

Stir-Fry Turkey

Whether done in traditional wok or a heavy skillet, a stir-fry is a quick and healthy meal. This recipe even makes use of leftover turkey!

Prep Time: 15 min
Servings: 4

Ingredients

1 Tbsp (15mL) coconut oil (or butter)

1 large garlic clove, minced

1 medium red onion, chopped

1 cup (90g) broccoli florets

1 medium carrot, cut in half-round slices

1 broccoli stem, peeled and sliced

1 Tbsp (15mL) tamari

2 cups (300g) celery sliced on the diagonal

2 medium kohlrabi, peeled and diced

2 cups (300g) cooked turkey (or chicken), cubed

2 tsp (10mL) dried thyme (or dried marjoram)

3 cups (90g) chopped kale (or spinach)

3 slices fresh gingerroot, minced

8 oz (230g) fresh mushrooms, sliced (or quartered)

¼ tsp (1.25mL) curry powder

Directions

Note: Prepare and have all ingredients close at hand before beginning to cook.

Heat coconut oil in a wok or heavy skillet over high heat. Add ginger and garlic; stir constantly for 30–45 seconds. Add onion, celery, carrot, broccoli stem, and kohlrabi and stir-fry, stirring constantly, for 3–4 minutes, or until vegetable colors brighten. Add broccoli flowerets, kale, and mushrooms, and continue to stir-fry for 1 minute. Add cooked turkey, thyme, and curry powder. Cover. Reduce heat to medium-low, and let steam continue the cooking for about 2 minutes.

Turn off heat. Stir in tamari, and serve immediately.

Variation: To use uncooked meat or poultry, add uniformly cut up pieces after the dense vegetables have been cooking for a couple of minutes.

Slow-Cooked Turkey Stew

This warm, welcoming one-dish-meal is perfect in fall or winter.

Prep Time: 15 min
Servings: 4

Ingredients

2 lb ((900g) turkey pieces

2 stalks celery, chopped

2 tsp (10mL) fresh thyme leaves

2 tsp (10mL) fresh oregano leaves

2 cups (400mL) water (or chicken stock)

1 medium leek, sliced

1 tsp (5mL) Spike (or Mrs. Dash) vegetable seasoning (or salt)

1 cup (150g) winter squash, peeled and cubed

1 medium carrot, chopped

1 stick cinnamon

1 cup (150g) cooked lentils

16 oz (450g) diced tomatoes (canned is fine)

Directions

Place turkey pieces, skin side down, in a slow cooker set on high, and sauté 3–5 minutes to release fat. Turn turkey, then add leek, celery, thyme, oregano, and Spike, and continue to sauté until leeks start to become translucent.

Add squash cubes, carrots, cinnamon, tomatoes, and water. Cover and simmer for 2–3 hours on high (or 6–8 hours on low).

A few minutes before serving, remove cinnamon stick and stir in cooked lentils.

Turkey Chili

Servings: 4

Ingredients

2 tsp (10mL) butter, divided

2 tsp (10mL) chili powder

1 lb (450g) lean ground turkey

1 cup (150g) coarsely chopped red bell pepper

1 medium onion, coarsely chopped (~¾ cup (120g)

1 bay leaf

1 clove garlic, minced

1 tsp (5mL) paprika

1 tsp (5mL) ground cumin

Dash ground cayenne pepper

14½ oz (400g) plum tomatoes, chopped (canned with juice is fine)

½ cup (120mL) chicken stock (or low-fat low-sodium chicken broth)

⅔ cup (100g) coarsely chopped celery (~⅔ stalk)

salt and freshly ground black pepper to taste

Directions

Heat 1 tsp (5mL) butter in a 3-quart saucepan over high heat. Add the turkey, and season to taste with the salt and black pepper. Break up the turkey and cook for 2–3 minutes, or until browned. Remove to a bowl and cover to keep warm.

Reduce the heat to low, heat the other 1 tsp butter, and cook the red pepper, onion, celery, and garlic for 3–5 minutes, or until vegetables begin to soften. Add the chili powder, paprika, cumin, and cayenne and cook, stirring, for 1 minute. Increase the heat to medium, and add the tomatoes, stock, and bay leaf. Bring to a boil over high heat. Reduce the heat to medium-low, and simmer uncovered for 15 minutes.

Add the browned turkey, and simmer 5 minutes more. Remove and discard the bay leaf before serving.

Herb-Roasted Turkey

Poultry

Prep Time: 20 min
Cook Time: 2-3 hours

Ingredients

1 12- to 14-lb turkey, brined

(see http://bbq.about.com/cs/
turkey/a/aa110103a.htm)

1 lemon, cut into wedges

1 cup (240mL) white wine

1 bay leaf

1 Tbsp (15mL) dried thyme

1 Tbsp (15mL) dried
rosemary

1 Tbsp (15mL) dried basil

3 sprigs fresh rosemary

3 sprigs fresh thyme

3–5 cups (700-1200mL)
chicken broth (enough to cover
the bottom of the pan ¼ inch)

4 Tbsp (60mL) unsalted
butter, softened

salt and cracked black
peppercorns to taste

¼–½ cup (60-120mL) olive
oil

Directions

Note: To create a golden skin,
uncover turkey and increase
oven temperature to 450°F
about 30 minutes before the
turkey is expected to be done.
Preheat oven to 325°F (163C)

Squeeze lemon juice over the
turkey. Place juiced lemon
wedges inside the chest cavity.
Mix olive oil, butter, salt,
and peppercorns, and rub
over the entire turkey. Place
fresh rosemary and thyme
underneath breast skin. Tie
legs together with kitchen
string, and close cavity. Pour
broth and wine in the bottom
of the roasting pan; add bay
leaf and dried herbs. Place
turkey, breast side up, on a
roasting rack in the pan, and
cover the pan.

Roast turkey until juices run
clear and a meat thermometer
reads 160°F (71C) when
inserted into the thickest
part of the breast without
touching the bone. (Estimate
15 minutes per pound; a 12- to
14-pound turkey should be
done in 2–3 hours.) Allow the
turkey to rest 20 minutes out
of the oven before carving.

www.BeyondDiet.com   - 269 -

Meat

Quick Beef Steaks with Mushrooms & Wine

Using cube steaks instead of the usual cuts can shorten cooking time and calories.

Prep Time: 10 min
Servings: 4

Ingredients

4 large (4- to 6-ounce) (112-168g) beef cube steaks

2 medium garlic cloves, minced

2 Tbsp (30mL) fresh parsley, finely chopped

2 Tbsp (30mL) butter

½ cup (120mL) red wine

8 oz (230g) fresh mushrooms, quartered

Directions

Place cube steaks in a quart-sized plastic bag, then set in a bowl to help bag stand up. Add wine, mushrooms, garlic, and parsley. Marinate mixture, refrigerated, for at least 30 minutes (to add flavor) and up to 24 hours (to tenderize the meat).

Melt butter in a large skillet over medium-high heat. Braise steaks, two at a time (reserving marinade for sauce), 2 minutes on each side. Remove steaks to serving platter and keep warm.

Pour reserved marinade into pan, and bring to a boil over medium-high heat. Cook for a couple of minutes, then pour over steaks. Serve immediately.

Variation: If you are short on time, simply heat marinade ingredients together in a small pan for 2–3 minutes while searing steaks in butter as directed. Remove steaks from pan. Deglaze pan and add to the warmed marinade. Pour over steaks.

Herb-Seasoned Steak Broil

This tasty center-of-the-plate dinner option is ready in minutes.

Prep Time: 10 min
Servings: 5

Ingredients

1 lb (450g) top-sirloin steak

1 tsp (5mL) ground celery seed

1 tsp (5mL) onion powder

1 tsp (5mL) coarse salt

2 tsp (10mL) coconut oil

2 Tbsp (30mL) Dijon-style mustard

2 tsp (10mL) grated horseradish (or prepared horseradish sauce)

2 tsp (10mL) dried thyme

½ tsp (2.5mL) freshly ground black pepper

Directions

Take steak out of refrigerator at least 30 minutes before cooking. Preheat oven to broil. Set oven rack 6 inches (15cm) from broiler unit.

Rub both sides of steak with coconut oil. Combine mustard and horseradish, and spread evenly on both sides of steak. Place steak on lightly greased broiler pan.

In small cup, mix thyme, celery seed, onion powder, salt, and pepper. Divide mixture, sprinkling half on each side of meat.

Broil steak for 3–4 minutes per side, or until browned. Remove steak to serving platter; let rest 1 minute. Slice and serve.

Grilled Cracked Pepper & Herb Steak

Cook Time: 20 min
Servings: 4

Ingredients

1 lb (450g) bone-in beef rib steak

1 Tbsp (15mL) garlic powder

1 Tbsp (15mL) dried rosemary, crushed

1 tsp (5mL) dried thyme

1 tsp (5mL) ground coriander

1 tsp (5mL) dried basil

1 tsp (5mL) dried oregano

2 tsp(10mL) olive oil

3 Tbsp (45mL) coarse salt

4 Tbsp (60mL) cracked black peppercorns

½ tsp (2.5mL) ground cayenne pepper (optional)

Directions

Rub steak with oil, and set aside on the counter for about 1 hour. (Bringing the steak to room temperature decreases grilling time and encourages even cooking.) Preheat grill to medium-high.

Combine salt, pepper, herbs, and cayenne (if using); coat the steak generously with this dry rub.

Sear steak 4–5 minutes per side for medium rare. Allow the steak to rest 5–10 minutes before carving for peak juiciness.

Garlic & Red Wine Filet Mignon

Prep Time: 25 min
Servings: 4

Ingredients

4 6-ounce (168g) filet mignon portions, each ~2 inches (5cm) thick

4 cloves garlic, thinly sliced

4 oz (113g) white mushrooms, thinly sliced

1 Tbsp (15mL) olive oil

½ cup (120mL) olive oil

¼ cup (60mL) balsamic vinegar

½ bottle red wine (cabernet sauvignon)

salt to taste

Directions

Slice into each filet lengthwise, creating a small pocket. Stuff each pocket with the equivalent of 1 clove of garlic, and season filets with salt. Mix olive oil and vinegar, and brush liberally over each filet.

Heat olive oil in a large skillet over medium-high heat. Sear filets for 2 minutes per side. Remove filets from skillet; add mushrooms and cook for 3–4 minutes, or until soft. Push mushrooms to the edges of the pan, and return filets. Add the wine, cover, and simmer for 10 minutes for filets that are medium done.

Roasted Garlic-Stuffed Rib Eyes

Prep Time: 30 min
Cook Time: 20 min
Servings: 4

Ingredients

2 8-ounce (230g) rib-eye steaks

2 whole heads garlic

4 tsp (20mL) olive oil

salt and freshly ground black pepper to taste

Directions

Preheat oven to 400°F (204C)

Rub each head of garlic with 1 tsp of olive oil, and place in a covered casserole dish. Bake for 15–20 minutes. Remove garlic from oven to cool, uncovered, but leave the oven on. Squeeze out roasted garlic; mash with a pinch each of salt and pepper.

Slice a 3-inch pocket lengthwise in each rib-eye steak. Fill each pocket with roasted garlic paste. Season both sides of each steak with salt and pepper.

Heat the remaining oil in an ovenproof skillet over medium-high heat. Sear steaks 3 minutes per side, then place in oven for 6 minutes for medium rare; add 1 or 2 minutes for each degree of doneness. Allow steaks to rest 10 minutes before serving.

Indian-Spiced Beef Burgers

Prep Time: 15 min
Cook Time: 15 min
Servings: 2

Ingredients

1 medium fresh jalapeño pepper, chopped

1 Tbsp (15mL) chopped fresh mint (or 1 tsp (5mL) crushed dried mint)

½ cup (90g) plain yogurt

⅓ cup (80g) chopped cucumber

¼ cup (40g) finely chopped onion

½ tsp (2.5mL) ground cumin

½ tsp (2.5mL) minced garlic (or ⅛ tsp (.125mL) garlic powder)

¼ tsp (1.25mL) salt

8 oz (230g) lean ground beef (or ground turkey)

Directions

Mix yogurt and cucumber in a small bowl. Refrigerate until ready to serve.

Preheat grill or broiler.

Combine onion, jalapeño, mint, cumin, garlic, and salt in a medium bowl, then add the ground beef. Mix all ingredients well. Form mixture into two ¾-inch (19mm) thick burgers.

Grill burgers over medium heat, uncovered, for 14–18 minutes (or 8–10 minutes if using turkey), turning once, or until meat is no longer pink. Top each burger with yogurt sauce, and serve.

Meat

Buffalo Chili

With this recipe, you'll discover that buffalo tastes a lot like beef—only better.

Prep Time: 15 min
Servings: 4

Ingredients

1 Tbsp (15mL) coconut oil

½ cup (75g) chopped onions

1½ cups (225g) chopped celery

1 cup (150g) chopped green bell pepper

1½ lb (675g) ground buffalo

2 tsp (10mL) dried thyme leaves

2 tsp (10mL) chili powder

2 tsp (10mL) ground cumin

2 medium garlic cloves, minced

1 tsp (5mL) salt

8 oz (150g) diced tomatoes (canned is fine)

12 oz (225g) (1 jar) prepared salsa

Directions

Melt coconut oil in a large skillet over medium-high heat. Sauté onions, garlic, celery, and green pepper 3–4 minutes, or until onion is translucent.

Add buffalo, thyme, chili powder, and cumin and cook for 5–6 minutes, stirring frequently.

Add salt, tomatoes, and salsa to pot. Cover, reduce heat, and simmer for a minimum of 1 hour.

Serve in bowls alone or over tiny steamed florets of cauliflower.

Buffalo Steaks with Red Pepper Sauce

A crust of crushed peppercorns, lemon, and salt and an easy sauce give these buffalo steaks a spicy kick.

Prep Time: 15 min
Servings: 4

Ingredients

4 cups (950mL) Chinese cabbage sliced on the diagonal into

¼-inch pieces

2–3 Tbsp (30-45mL) whole green and black peppercorns

1 tsp (5mL) coarse salt

1 tsp (5mL) lemon zest

1 lb (450g) buffalo rib-eye steaks

1 tsp (5mL) coconut oil (or butter)

1 tsp (5mL) tamari (or Spike vegetable seasoning)

1 medium garlic clove, minced

1 pinch salt

8 oz (226g) roasted red peppers (jarred are fine)

Directions

Crush peppercorns with the back of a spoon, with a mortar and pestle, or in a spice grinder; mix with coarse salt and lemon zest. Season both sides of the steaks with this mixture, then set them aside to marinate for up to 30 minutes.

Sear steaks by broiling, grilling, or frying in heavy cast-iron skillet over medium-high heat, 3 minutes per side. Set aside steaks and keep warm.

In a heavy cast-iron skillet, heat 1 tsp coconut oil over high heat, then stir-fry Chinese cabbage and garlic with a pinch of salt until cabbage is wilted.

Meanwhile, blend roasted red peppers in blender with tamari.

To assemble, pile serving platter with braised cabbage, top with steaks, and pour red pepper sauce over top. Serve immediately.

Horseradish Buffalo Burgers

This recipe goes nicely with Asparagus with Sesame Seeds (page 14) and a salad.

Prep Time: 10 min
Servings: 4

Ingredients

1 lb (400g) ground buffalo

2 Tbsp (30mL) prepared horseradish

½ tsp (2.5mL) Spike vegetable seasoning (or salt)

3–4 grinds black pepper

Directions

Mix the ground meat with the remaining ingredients. Form into patties.

Broil in the oven, grill, or fry in a hot cast-iron skillet over medium-high heat, 3–4 minutes on a side, until browned. Do not overcook. Serve immediately.

Roasted Leg of Lamb (or Chevon)

Servings: 4-6

Ingredients

1 6- to 8-lb (2700g-3600g) leg of lamb (or chevon [baby goat])

1 Tbsp (15mL) minced fresh rosemary

1 clove garlic, slivered

1 1-inch (2.5cm) piece of fresh gingerroot, peeled and minced

2 Tbsp (30mL) olive oil

½ cup (120mL) Dijon-style mustard

¼ cup (60mL) soy sauce

Directions

Preheat oven to 350°F (177C)

Blend mustard, soy sauce, rosemary, garlic, and ginger in a bowl. Whisk in oil to make a creamy mixture, then set aside the sauce.

Make four shallow slashes in the lamb with a sharp knife; tuck a sliver of garlic into each. Brush the lamb liberally with sauce, and let stand on the counter for 1–2 hours.

Roast lamb on a rack for 1¼ to 1½ hours, or until a meat thermometer reads 150°F (66C) (medium doneness). Allow the roast to rest for at least 15 minutes before carving; the temperature will increase to about 160°F (71C) as it rests.

Herbed Lemony Lamb Chops

The lemony seasoning makes delicious lamb chops, whichever cut you prefer.

Prep Time: 30-35 min
Servings: 4

Ingredients

4 lamb shoulder chops

3 Tbsp (45mL) lemon juice

2 Tbsp (30mL) butter

1 tsp (5mL) lemon zest (or ½ (2.5mL) tsp lemon pepper seasoning)

1 tsp (5mL) dried oregano

1 tsp (5mL) dried tarragon

1 Tbsp (15mL) soy sauce

½ tsp (2.5mL) dried rosemary, crushed

Directions

Combine lemon zest, herbs, lemon juice, and soy sauce in a small bowl; set aside.

Heat butter in a large skillet over medium-high heat. Brown lamb chops on both sides, and leave in skillet. Pour seasoning over chops in skillet. Cover, and simmer over medium-low heat for 20–25 minutes, or until chops are tender.

Variation: The same seasoning ingredients could be used on lamb loin chops to be broiled. Reduce the amount of lemon juice to 1 Tbsp and mix with herbs to make a paste. Spread on loin chops and broil 3–4 minutes per side, depending up thickness. Do not overcook.

Meat

Venison Stew

Venison is low in fat and especially good in stews, where it is cooked in liquid.

Prep Time: 15 min
Servings: 6

Ingredients

1½ lb (675g) stewing venison

1 pinch salt

1 pinch freshly ground black pepper

1 Tbsp (15mL) coconut oil (or butter)

1 medium red onion, sliced

1 tsp (5mL) ground cinnamon

1 tsp (5mL) orange zest

2 tsp (10mL) dried thyme

3 stalks celery, sliced on the diagonal

3 medium kohlrabi, peeled and chopped

3 cups (700mL) beef stock

½ cup (75g) fresh cranberries

Directions

Season venison with salt and pepper.

Heat coconut oil in large stockpot or Dutch oven over medium heat. Sauté onion and celery until onion starts to become translucent. Remove and set aside vegetables.

Add venison to pan, and sear until browned on all sides. Stir in thyme, cinnamon, orange zest, cranberries, kohlrabi, and stock. Return the sautéed vegetables to the pan.

Heat the mixture until it starts to bubble, cover, and lower heat to medium-low. Simmer for 45–50 minutes, or until venison is tender.

Meat

Grilled Pork Tenderloin with Rosemary-Mustard Rub

Pork is easy to prepare and offers a flavorful alternative to chicken.

(Wild Oats Marketplace online recipes)

Prep Time: 15 min
Marinate Time: 30 min
Cook Time: 15-20 min
Servings: 4

Ingredients

4 sprigs fresh rosemary

2–3 cloves garlic, peeled

3 Tbsp (45mL) olive oil

2 tsp (10mL) coarse salt

2 tsp (10mL) cracked black peppercorns

2 Tbsp (30mL) stone-ground mustard

1 lb (450g) pork tenderloin, trimmed

Directions

Strip rosemary leaves from stems and place in a small food processor bowl with garlic, oil, salt, pepper, and mustard. Pulse the mixture to make a paste.

Smooth the paste over the pork, place on a baking sheet, cover, and place in the refrigerator for 30 minutes. Preheat gas grill to high. Brush grate with olive oil. Sear pork for 3 minutes per side. Reduce heat to medium-low, cover, and cook pork for 8–10 minutes, or until the internal temperature reaches 145°F (63C). Transfer pork to a platter. Let rest for 6–8 minutes before slicing and serving.

Variation: Try the rosemary–mustard rub on turkey breast, a whole roasting chicken, or a fish fillet.

Marinated Pork Chops

(Wild Oats Marketplace online recipes)

Servings: 6

Ingredients

6 pork chops, each ~¾ inch (19mm) thick

2 cloves garlic, minced

3 tsp (15mL) paprika

salt and freshly ground black pepper to taste

1 cup (240mL) white wine

Directions

Place pork chops in one layer in a shallow ovenproof baking dish. Combine garlic, paprika, salt, and pepper, and spread over chops. Pour the white wine over all. Cover and refrigerate for 6 hours. Preheat oven to 300°F (150C) Uncover the dish and bake chops uncovered in the marinade for 1 hour.

Meat

Veal Chops
(Sally Fallon, *Nourishing Traditions*)

Servings: 4

Ingredients

4 veal chops

juice of 1 lemon

½ tsp (2.5mL) dried thyme

2 Tbsp (30mL) butter

2 Tbsp (30mL) olive oil

½ cup (120mL) dry white wine (or vermouth)

2 cups (480mL) beef stock

Directions

Marinate the veal chops for several hours in lemon juice mixed with thyme.

Dry chops thoroughly. Heat the butter and oil in a heavy skillet, and brown the chops, two at a time, on both sides. Remove chops to a plate. Discard the browning oil from the skillet, and add wine and stock. Bring the mixture to a rapid boil, stirring to scrape up accumulated veal juices. Skim sauce, and return the chops to the skillet. Reduce heat to a simmer, cover, and cook about 30 minutes, or until chops are tender.

Remove chops to a heated platter and keep warm. Bring the liquid to a rapid boil, and skim occasionally until sauce thickens. Spoon sauce over chops to serve.

Fish

Easy Broiled Halibut

Servings: 6-8

Ingredients

2 lb (900g) center-cut halibut steak

salt (or Herbamare seasoned salt) to taste

freshly ground black pepper to taste

¼ cup (60mL) (or more if desired) lemon juice

1 Tbsp (15mL) butter (or coconut oil)

Directions

Wipe halibut with a damp cloth. Season with salt, pepper, and lemon juice, and dot with butter. Broil, turning frequently, till brown.

Mustard-Crusted Halibut

Serve on a bed of baby spinach, arugula, and water chestnuts.

Servings: 1-2

Ingredients

6 oz (168g) center-cut halibut steak

1 tsp (5mL) whole-grain mustard

1 tsp (5mL) chopped fresh thyme

1 Tbsp (15mL) chopped fresh oregano

1 tsp (5mL) chopped fresh rosemary

1 tsp (5mL) water

1–2 Tbsp (15-30mL) butter

½ tsp (2.5mL) freshly ground black pepper

Directions

Preheat oven to 350°F (176C)

In a small bowl, combine the mustard, thyme, oregano, rosemary, pepper, and water and blend well to make a paste.

Butter an ovenproof baking dish. Place halibut in the dish and spread with the mustard–herb paste. Bake for 15–20 minutes, or until fish flakes easily with a fork.

Grilled Swordfish

Servings: 6

Ingredients

1½ lb (675g) swordfish steaks

¾ cup (180mL) Cilantro Marinade (page 232)

1 cup (237mL) Béarnaise Sauce (page 234)

Directions

Brush both sides of the swordfish with Cilantro Marinade, cover, and marinate in the refrigerator for several hours.

Broil or grill swordfish for 5–10 minutes per side, depending on the thickness of the steaks. Be careful not to let the swordfish burn. Serve topped with Béarnaise Sauce.

Easy Smothered Salmon

Servings: 6

Ingredients

2 Tbsp (30mL) coconut oil (or butter)

2 slices turkey bacon, chopped

1 tsp (5mL) salt

1–2 Tbsp (15-30mL) butter

2 cups (300g) canned salmon

½ cup (120mL) boiling water

¾ cup (76g) diced celery

¾ cup (76g) chopped onion

Directions

Preheat oven to 375°F (190C)

Melt oil in a heavy skillet. Add oil, bacon, celery, onion, and salt and fry until celery and onion are light brown.

Butter a covered ovenproof baking dish, and place salmon in center. Arrange vegetable mixture around salmon. Add water and cover.

Bake for 30 minutes. Remove cover and bake another 10 minutes.

Salmon with Pecan Pesto

Servings: 4

Ingredients

5 oz (140g) shelled pecans

4 salmon fillets **(1½ lb (675g) total)**

3 oz (85g) cold butter, cut into ½-Tbsp (2.5mL) pats

2–3 fresh jalapeño peppers, seeded and coarsely chopped

1 3-inch (7.6cm) sprig of rosemary

1 Tbsp (15mL) olive oil

salt and freshly ground black pepper to taste

zest of ½ small lemon (or small orange), finely chopped

Directions

Preheat oven to 300°F (150C)

Toast pecans on a cookie sheet about 20–30 minutes, or until they release their aroma. Set aside to cool.

Strip rosemary leaves from stems, mince, and set aside.

Rinse salmon and pat dry. Butterfly fillets with a sharp knife, if desired. Rub salmon with olive oil; season with salt and pepper. Heat heavy skillet over medium heat. Pan-fry fillets until firm to the touch.

Place the toasted pecans, rosemary, butter, jalapeños, and lemon zest in a food processor. Process for 5–8 seconds, scrape the bowl, and repeat two or three times until a paste (pesto) forms. Do not overprocess.

Spread the pesto over the cooked salmon, and serve immediately.

Baked Herbed Salmon

A traditional Mediterranean pesto makes an low-carbohydrate salmon dish that's quick, elegant, and tasty. The fish bakes with the sauce while you prepare the rest of the meal.

Prep Time: 10 min
Servings: 4

Ingredients

4 6-ounce (168g) salmon fillets

2 medium garlic cloves, coarsely chopped

2 tsp (10mL) lemon zest

1 Tbsp (15mL) capers (or green olives)

1 cup (30g) coarsely chopped flat-leaf Italian parsley

1 cup (30g) coarsely chopped cilantro leaves

1 Tbsp (15mL) olive oil

1 tsp (5mL) ground cumin

½ tsp (2.5mL) Spike vegetable seasoning (or salt)

½ tsp (2.5mL) freshly ground black pepper

5 oz (30mL) fresh lemon juice

salt and freshly ground black pepper to taste

Directions

Preheat oven to 350°F.

Rinse salmon and place on lightly greased cookie sheet or in an ovenproof baking dish. Season with salt and pepper.

In food processor, process olive oil, garlic, Spike, cumin, pepper, capers, parsley, cilantro, lemon zest, and lemon juice until well combined. Pour sauce over fish.

Bake for 13–15 minutes, or until salmon flakes easily with a fork.

Broiled Lemon Salmon

Fresh lemon juice is the key to making broiled salmon exceptional.

Servings: 4

Ingredients

4 6-ounce (168g) salmon fillets
2 Tbsp (30mL) chopped chives
1 Tbsp (15mL) tamari
1 clove garlic, minced
1 whole lemon, cut into ⅛-inch (3mm) slices
1 tsp (5mL) olive oil
⅓ cup (20mL) fresh lemon juice

Directions

Whisk tamari, garlic, lemon juice, olive oil, and chives. Pour over fillets, and marinate with lemon slices, turning occasionally, for 20–30 minutes.

Broil salmon (with lemon slices around broiling pan) with rack set 6 inches (15cm) beneath broiler unit for 3–4 minutes. Turn salmon carefully, and continue to broil another 3 minutes, or until fillets are brown and flake easily with a fork.

Remove salmon to a serving platter. Place broiled lemon slices on top of fish. Pour any remaining marinade over. Serve immediately.

Salmon Ceviche

In South America, Japan, and elsewhere, marinated raw fish is served as an appetizer. It is a popular way to preserve the flavor, nutrition, and digestibility of fresh fish. Serve with butter lettuce or other leafy salad greens.

Prep Time: 10 min
Servings: 4

Ingredients

1 lb (450g) salmon

1 cup (150g) chopped tomatoes

1 cup (237mL) fresh lime juice

2 Tbsp (30mL) seeded and finely chopped serrano pepper (or 1 chili pepper, minced)

2 tsp (10mL) salt

2 cups (32g) chopped cilantro (or parsley)

⅓ cup (53g) finely diced red onion

Directions

Skin salmon, and chop into ¼- to ½-inch(6-13mm) pieces. Combine salmon, onion, lime juice, hot pepper, and salt. Marinate for several hours or overnight.

About 10–15 minutes before serving, add chopped tomatoes and cilantro to salmon mixture, and stir to combine.

Beans

Cooked Beans

This is a great way to have delicious cooked beans ready at any moment to heat and eat or add to a recipe. Cook your favorite bean with the following indications.

Prep Time: Varies
Cook Time: Varies
Servings: 4-6

Ingredients

1 cup (150g) dried beans (any variety)

Directions

Sort and clean the dried beans. Soak the beans in boiling water for 1 - 2 hours, or 6 - 12 hours in cold water, until they're doubled in size and wrinkle free - soaking time varies with the bean. Drain and rinse the soaked beans, place in medium saucepan, cover with cold unsalted water. Bring to boil uncovered, boil for ten minutes. Skim the foam off the beans with a ladle or large flat spoon. Cover and simmer the beans for 1 - 2 hours OR cook 8 minutes at high pressure in a pressure cooker.

Slow cooker or crockpot: Add the beans, cover and turn the heat to low. Cooking time will vary with the bean, but six hours in the crockpot on low is about right for pinto beans

Note: It's always worthwhile to double the bean recipe, and freeze in small containers or freezer bags for future vegetarian or vegan bean recipes.

Homemade Hummus

Prep Time: 10 min
Makes: 2 cups

Ingredients

1 (15.5 ounce) (450g) can garbanzo beans (chickpeas), drained

1/3 cup (50g) pitted Spanish Manzanilla olives

1 tsp (5mL) minced garlic

1 ½ tsps (7.5mL) chopped fresh basil

1 tsp (5mL) cilantro leaves

2 Tbsp (30mL) lemon juice

3 Tbsp (45mL) olive oil

salt and pepper to taste

Directions

Place garbanzo beans, olives, and garlic into the bowl of a blender or food processor. Pour in olive oil and lemon juice; season with basil, cilantro, salt, and pepper. Cover and puree until smooth. Hummus can be served immediately, or covered, and stored in the refrigerator until ready to use.

Kidney Bean & Mushroom Veggie Burger

Prep Time: 1 hour
Cook Time: 12 min
Servings: 4-6

Ingredients

2 medium carrots

1 cup (90g) oats

1 14 ounce (400g) can kidney beans, drained

½ cup (75g) mushrooms

½ onion

½ red or yellow bell pepper

1 egg

2 Tbsp (30mL) organic ketchup (optional as it adds sugar)

½ tsp (2.5mL) garlic salt

Directions

Process carrot in food processor until grated. Add oats and beans and pulse a few times.

Add remaining ingredients and process until well combined but still slightly coarse.

Chill for at least 45 minutes then form into 4 - 6 patties. Broil for 5-6 minutes on each side. You could also cook these mushroom veggie burgers on the grill, or pan fry in coconut oil.

Black Bean Veggie Burgers

Prep Time: 15 min
Cooking Time: 20-30 min
Servings: 10

Ingredients

2 cups (300g) black beans cooked

½ cup (75g) green pepper, chopped fine

½ cup (75g) red onion, chopped fine

1 large stalk celery, chopped fine

2 -4 cloves garlic minced (depends how much you like garlic)

1 tsp (5mL) cumin

1 Tbsp (15mL) cooking oil

¼ tsp (1.25mL) cayenne pepper

Salt and pepper to taste

1/3 cup (60g) hummus

½ cup (45g) rolled oats

Directions

2 slices sprouted grain or spelt bread crumbled into tiny pieces (hint: blender or food processor works great)

Mash or puree half the beans, add reserved beans and all other ingredients EXCEPT hummus. Mix well by hand. Add enough of the hummus or other liquid ingredient to moisten mixture fairly well. Mixture may seem a little sticky, but it's better than a bit dry, because they WILL dry out while cooking. Cook on medium until brown, approx. 10 - 15 min per side. Fantastic with a little brown mustard or horseradish.

Garbanzo Bean Burger

Prep Time: 45 min
Cook Time: 30 min
Servings: 4

Ingredients

1 (15 ounce) (450g) can garbanzo beans, rinsed and drained

1 red bell pepper, finely chopped

1 carrot, grated

1 tsp (5mL) olive oil (optional)

1 red chile pepper, seeded and minced

1 Tbsp (15mL) tahini paste

2 Tbsp (30mL) chopped fresh cilantro

3 cloves garlic, minced

salt and black pepper to taste

Directions

Place garbanzo beans in the food processor with bell pepper, carrot, garlic, red chile pepper, cilantro, tahini, salt, and pepper. Pulse 5 times, scrape the sides, and pulse again until the mixture is evenly mixed. If the mixture looks dry, add olive oil. Refrigerate mixture for 30 minutes. Preheat oven to 350 degrees F (175 degrees C). Prepare baking sheet with parchment paper or lightly grease with coconut oil. Shape the mixture into patties. Bake for 20 minutes, then carefully flip burgers and bake 10 more minutes, or until brown.

Veggie Vegetarian Chili

You can freeze this chili and keep it on hand to reheat for a quick and easy lunch or dinner solution.

Cooking Time: 30 min
Servings: 16

Ingredients

3 cloves garlic, minced

2 Tbsp (30mL) chili powder

1 Tbsp (15mL) butter or coconut oil

1 cup (150g) chopped onion

1 cup chopped (150g) carrots

1 cup chopped (150g) green bell pepper

1 cup chopped (150g) red bell pepper

1 ½ cups (225g) chopped fresh mushrooms

1 (28 oz) (950mL) can whole peeled tomatoes with liquid, chopped

1 (15 oz) (475mL) can black beans, undrained

1 (15 oz) (475mL) can kidney beans, undrained

1 (15 oz) (475mL) can pinto beans, undrained

1 Tbsp (15mL) cumin

1 ½ Tbsp (22.5mL) dried oregano

1 ½ Tbsp (22.5mL) dried basil

½ Tbsp (7.5mL) garlic powder

Directions

Heat the butter or coconut oil in a large pot over medium heat. Cook and stir the garlic, onion, and carrots in the pot until tender. Mix in the green bell pepper and red bell pepper. Season with chili powder. Continue cooking 5 minutes, or until peppers are tender. Mix the mushrooms into the pot. Stir in the tomatoes with liquid, black beans with liquid, kidney beans with liquid, and pinto beans with liquid. Season with cumin, oregano, basil, and garlic powder. Bring to a boil. Reduce heat to medium, cover, and cook 20 minutes, stirring occasionally.

Lentil and Vegetable Soup

Prep Time: 30 min
Cook Time: 1 1/2 - 2 hours
Servings: 6

Ingredients

3 carrots, chopped

2 cups (300g) shredded cabbage

2 cups (480mL) chicken broth

1 cup (150g) chopped onion

1 stalk celery, chopped

1 (28 oz) (950mL) can whole peeled tomatoes, chopped

1 clove garlic, crushed

½ cup (120mL) red or green lentils

1 tsp (5mL) Celtic Sea salt

½ tsp (2.5mL) ground black pepper

½ tsp (2.5mL) dried basil

½ tsp (2.5mL) dried thyme

¼ tsp (1.25mL) curry powder

Directions

Place the lentils into a stockpot or a Dutch oven and add water to twice the depth of the lentils. Bring to a boil, then lower heat and let simmer for about 15 minutes. Drain and rinse lentils; return them to the pot. Add onion, celery, cabbage, tomatoes, chicken broth, carrots and garlic to the pot and season with salt, pepper, sugar, basil, thyme and curry. Cook, simmering for 1 ½ to 2 hours or until desired tenderness is achieved.

Beans

Slow Cooker Lentil Rice Soup

Dried lentils and uncooked brown rice are combined with vegetables, seasonings and broth in this easy and nutritious soup. Chopped mushrooms are added in the last of the 8 hours of cooking time.

Prep Time: 20 min
Cooking Time: 7-8 hours
Servings: 11

Ingredients

2 cups (300g) dry lentils

2 cups (380g) uncooked long grain brown rice

1 cup (150g) chopped carrots

1 cup (150g) sliced fresh mushrooms

1 cup (240mL) vegetable broth

1 Tbsp (15mL) salt

1 tsp (5mL) garlic powder

½ cup (75g) chopped celery

½ onion, chopped

½ tsp (2.5mL) ground black pepper

8 cups (1920mL) water

Directions

Place all ingredients except the mushrooms in the slow cooker and cook on low for 7 to 8 hours. Stir in the mushrooms 1 hour before serving.

Pinto Bean Soup

Prep Time: 20 min
Cook Time: 30 min
Servings: 4-6

Ingredients

3 Tbsp (45mL) olive oil

2 stalks celery

2 thin slices raw ginger, peeled, or ½ tsp (2.5mL) dried, if you don't have fresh

2 cups (300g) cooked pinto beans (OR 2 cans)

2 cups (480mL) water

2 tsp (10mL) dry basil leaves OR 2 Tbsp (30mL) minced fresh

1 large yam or small butternut squash

1 jalapeno pepper, seeded. If you don't have it, use a pinch of cayenne

1 - 2 cloves garlic

1 tsp (5mL) brown mustard seed

1 tsp (5mL) paprika

1 tsp (5mL) ground coriander seed

1 Tbsp (15mL) gluten-free soy sauce

2/3 cup (160mL) coconut milk

½ tsp (2.5mL) ground cumin seed

½ head of cauliflower

½ tsp (2.5mL) turmeric

½ tsp (2.5mL) fennel

½ cinnamon stick

½ tsp (2.5mL) salt or to taste

½ tsp (2.5mL) fresh ground pepper or to taste

¼ cup (60mL) chopped fresh parsley leaves

1 bay leaf

Directions

Combine pinto beans, water, coconut milk, bay leaf, cinnamon stick, and veggie cube, heat on low Heat oil on low in a large sauté pan.

Mince the fresh jalapeno, ginger, and garlic. Peel and cut the yam in 1 inch (2.5cm) dice. Wash and thinly slice the celery. Remove stem and leaves from ½ head of cauliflower, cut in bite-sized pieces and set aside. Add all the veggies except cauliflower to the oil, plus the mustard seeds. Turn the heat up a bit and sauté for about ten minutes. Add the cauliflower and the remaining spices, and stir-fry for a few minutes. Add the beans and 2 cups (480mL) water and coconut milk, then cover and simmer on low until veggies are tender, and soup has thickened, about 20 minutes, stirring several times. Chop the parsley and add with salt, pepper and soy sauce to taste.

Lima Bean Stew

Prep Time: Varies
Cooking Time: 6-8 hours
Servings: 6-8

Ingredients

2 large carrots, peeled and diced

2 ginger slices, peeled

2 celery sticks, chopped in ¼ inch slices

2 bay leaves

2 Tbsp olive oil

1 small cauliflower, cut in large pieces

1 ½ cups dry lima beans

1 tsp thyme leaves

1 tsp salt

½ tsp turmeric

½ tsp ground cumin

¼ cup minced fresh parsley
pinch cayenne or to taste

Fresh ground pepper to taste

Directions

Soak the lima beans in 2 qt cold water, overnight or up to twelve hours. Preheat the crockpot on high. Add the lima beans to a saucepan, with water to cover. Bring them to a boil. Prep the veggies and add to the crockpot with lima beans and cooking water

Add more water if needed to cover. Add the bay leaves, ginger slices, and thyme. Reduce heat to low, cover and cook for 6 - 8 hours. Heat the oil on low in a small frying pan. Add the cumin, coriander, turmeric & cayenne. Heat gently for a few minutes. Using a spatula, transfer spices and oil to the crockpot. Add ¼ cup minced parsley, salt and pepper to taste. Stir gently, cover and cook for another 15 minutes. Remove the ginger slices and bay leaves when serving.

Beans

Quinoa Red Lentil Stew

Prep Time: 15 min
Cook Time: Varies
Servings: 4-6

Ingredients

4 green cardamom pods

4 Tbsp (60mL) minced fresh herbs: parsley, cilantro or basil

2 thin slices fresh ginger

2 bay leaves

2 large carrots

2 stalks celery

2 inch (5cm) piece cinnamon stick

1 small head cauliflower

1 tsp (5mL) salt or to taste

½ cup (75g) quinoa

¾ cup (110g) small red lentils (masoor dhal)

½ tsp (2.5mL) ground cumin

½ tsp (2.5mL) ground fennel seed

½ tsp (2.5mL) turmeric

6 cups (1440mL) water

For a spicier flavor, Add ½ - 1 tsp (2.5-5mL) green curry paste OR ¼ tsp (1.25mL) cayenne powder

Directions

Rinse the quinoa and red lentils in a bowl or pan, then drain into a colander. Peel the carrots, slice lengthwise, then slice in thin pieces. Wash and trim the celery stalks, then slice crosswise in thin pieces. Break or cut the cauliflower into large chunks - these will break up into smaller pieces as they cook. Combine quinoa, lentils, cumin, fennel, turmeric, bay leaves, cinnamon stick, cardamom pods and fresh ginger slices in the crockpot, and cover with the 6 cups water. Cover and cook on low for 6 hours or more if needed. Just before serving, add the minced fresh herb, and optional greens

When serving, remove the ginger slices, bay leaves, cinnamon stick, and cardamom pods, as you come across them. If you don't have a crockpot, you can make this quinoa recipe on the stove. Bring to a boil, cover and cook on low heat for 20 - 30 min.

Black Bean Dip

A spicy black bean paste that works great as a dip, in burritos, or on nachos.

Prep Time: 10 min
Cook Time: 10 min
Makes: 2 cups

Ingredients

2 cups (300g) black beans, canned and drained or soaked and

cooked (link to cooked beans recipe)

2-3 limes, juiced

1 Tbsp (15mL) olive oil

1 tsp (5mL) ground coriander

1 tsp (5mL) ground cumin

1 tsp (5mL) chipotle chile, puréed OR ½ t (2.5mL) cayenne

½ cup (120mL) hot water

¼ cup (40g) scallions, sliced

¼ cup (60mL) cilantro, chopped

½-1 tsp (2.5-5mL) salt

Directions

Place the beans in the food processor or bowl, pour water over them, and let sit.

Meanwhile, heat the oil over low - medium heat, add the scallions, coriander, and cumin, and sauté, stirring frequently, until tender, about 10 minutes.

Add spice mixture, cilantro, and chile to the beans and purée until chunky, 10-20 seconds. Add lime juice and salt, mix, taste, and add more chile/cayenne, lime juice, and salt as needed.

Bean dip keeps in refrigerator for up to 5 days, but it tastes best warm or at room temperature.

Cashew Chili

Cashew chili is easy, delicious, filling, and vegetarian. What more can you ask for?

Prep Time: 10 min
Cook Time: 10 min
Servings: 4

Ingredients

1 **Tbsp (15mL)** olive oil

1 stalk celery

1 **tsp (5mL)** black pepper

1 **tsp (5mL)** minced basil

1 **tsp (5mL)** minced oregano

1 green bell pepper

1 bay leaf

1-2 Tbsp (15-30mL) cider vinegar

1-2 cans kidney beans, in water

2 medium onions

2 cups (480g) canned tomatoes, with juice

½-1 Tbsp (2.5-5mL) chili powder

¼ tsp (1.25mL) cumin

½-1 (75-150g) cup cashews

Directions

Chop the celery, onions, and bell pepper, then sauté them in olive oil until tender.

Add tomatoes and beans (with water) and all spices. Cover and simmer for 5-10 minutes, until you're happy with the amount of liquid. Add vinegar and cashews.

Taste and adjust seasonings, remove bay leaf, and serve. For a soupier consistency, use less beans and nuts.

Beans

Dal

Dal is the Indian term for lentils, and in cooking refers to any of the many Indian dishes made with lentils. There are many variations ranging from simple to complex. This recipe is on the easy side.

Prep Time: 10 min
Cook Time: 40 min
Makes: 2 cups

Ingredients

1 cup (150g) red lentils (masoor dal) or brown lentils

1 small onion, minced

1 chile, seeded and chopped

1 dried red chile, crumbled OR ¼ t (1.25mL) red pepper flakes

1 tsp (5mL) mustard seeds

½ tsp (2.5mL) turmeric

2 cloves garlic, sliced

2 shallots, diced

3 Tbsp (45mL) butter or olive oil

3 bay leaves

3 cups (700mL) water

15 oz (420mL) can unsweetened coconut milk

salt

Directions

Wash the lentils thoroughly and drain well.

Heat 2 Tbsp (30g) butter over medium-high heat, then sauté onion, garlic, and chile for 1 minute. Add lentils, turmeric, and 3 c (700mL) water. Bring to a boil, lower heat, cover, and simmer until lentils are soft, about 30 minutes.

Remove the cream from the top of the coconut milk and reserve for some other use. Add coconut milk to lentils and simmer, stirring occasionally, for 5 minutes. Add a bit of salt, taste, and remove from heat.
Heat remaining 1 Tbsp butter over high heat. Add remaining ingredients and sauté about 1 minute, until mustard seeds turn grey. Stir into lentils and serve.

White Bean and Tomato Soup

This white bean and tomato soup flavored with sage and thyme is an elegant alternative to minestrone soup.

Prep Time: 8 hours
Cook Time: 1-1 1/2 hours
Servings: 4-6

Ingredients

1 tsp (5mL) salt

1 medium onion, chopped

1 pound (450g) fresh tomatoes or **2 c (300g)** canned tomatoes, chopped, or **2 c (475mL)** plain tomato sauce

½ cup (75g) dry whitebeans, washed and soaked for at least 8 hours

3 bay leaves

3 Tbsp (45mL) olive oil

4 cloves garlic, peeled

6 branches of thyme or **¼ t (1.25mL)** dried thyme

8 cups (1920mL) water

10 sage leaves or **1 tsp (5mL)** dried sage

Directions

Drain and rinse the beans and place in pot along with water, 5 sage leaves, 2 bay leaves, thyme, 3 whole cloves garlic, and 1 Tbsp (15mL) oil. Bring to a boil, add ½ t (2.5mL) salt, lower heat, and simmer about an hour, until beans just tender.

Set the colander over a bowl; strain the beans; and remove the garlic, bay leaves, and thyme stems. Set both the cooking water and beans aside.

Heat remaining oil along as you mince the last garlic clove. Add to pot along with the remaining sage and bay leaf. Sauté a minute or two, add onion, and cook, stirring frequently, for 8-10 minutes, until soft. Add the tomatoes, cooking liquid, and remaining salt, bring to a boil, and simmer for 20 minutes. Then add beans and cook another 10 minutes.

Serve hot or set aside to cool, then refrigerate in an airtight container - the flavor will actually improve over the next day or two.

Shepherd's Pie

This vegetarian shepherd's pie recipe is a simple yet delicious lambless version of the real thing.

Prep Time: 30 min
Cook Time: 30 min
Makes: 6

Ingredients

1 large tomato, chopped

1 cup (240mL) vegetable stock or water

1 tsp (5mL) gluten-free soy sauce

2½ Tbsp (37.5mL) olive oil

2 cloves garlic, minced

2 to 2½ cups (300-375g) mashed cauliflower

3 cups (450g) mixed vegetables, finely chopped

3 cups (450g) cooked legumes

½ cup (75g) onion, minced

pepper

Directions

Heat 2 Tbsp (30mL) oil over medium heat, add garlic, and sauté for 2 minutes. Add onion and continue sautéing until soft, about 5 minutes. Add tomato and cook for two more minutes, stirring frequently. (If you need to make the mashed potatoes, start them now). Add stock and vegetables, bring to boil, cover, lower heat, and cook until vegetables are tender, about 5-10 minutes. Add soy sauce and pepper, taste, and adjust seasonings as necessary.

Preheat oven to 350F (177C). Use remaining ½ Tbsp oil to grease pie plate. Arrange vegetables in it, then cover with a layer of mashed potatoes. Garnish.

Bake until bubbly, about 30 minutes. Serve hot.

Chickpea Mock Tuna Salad

A vegetarian "tuna" salad made with chickpeas, almonds, and seeds. While this doesn't take exactly like tuna salad, it's close enough and delicious.

Prep Time: 24 hours
Cook Time: 45 min
Servings: 4

Ingredients

½ cup (75g) almonds

½ cup (75g) sunflower seeds

¼ cup (40g) sesame seeds

½ cup (120g) homemade mayonnaise

1/3 cup (50g) red onion, minced

several cups of water

1 Tbsp (15mL) water (can be from chickpea cooking water)

1 Tbsp (15mL) gluten-free soy sauce

1 cup (240g) soaked and cooked or canned chickpeas, drained and

rinsed

1-2 tsp (5-10mL) kelp powder

1 stalk celery, minced

2 Tbsp (30mL) lemon juice

2 tsp (10mL) flaxseed or olive oil

2 Tbsp (30mL) fresh parsley, minced

Directions

Rinse the almonds and seeds (a sieve or fine-holed colander is needed for the sesame seeds), place in bowl, cover with water, and let soak overnight. Rinse and drain.

Place the almonds, seeds, chickpeas, lemon juice, T water, soy sauce, oil, and kelp powder in food processor. Blend until well mixed but not quite smooth, 1-2 minutes.

Combine the mayonnaise, celery, onion, and parsley in the bowl, then add chickpea mixture. Cover and refrigerate for at least 30 minutes.

This mock tuna salad will last 2-3 days in the refrigerator.

Eggs

Spanish Tortilla

This potato omelette is a traditional Spanish tapa, or appetizer, but it's equally good for breakfast or brunch.

Prep Time: 15 min
Cook Time: 15 min
Servings: 6

Ingredients

1 pound (450g) potatoes (preferably sweet potatoes), peeled

1 large onion, diced

¼ cup (60mL) olive oil

5 eggs

salt and pepper

Directions

Slice the potatoes as thin as possible and dry with a paper towel. Sauté potatoes and onions in olive oil over medium heat, turning frequently, until golden brown (about three minutes).

Meanwhile, beat the eggs with salt and pepper until foamy, 1-2 minutes. Pour the eggs over the potatoes, cover, lower the heat, and cook for about 5-7 minutes, until the omelette is set and the bottom is golden brown. Slide the omelette onto a plate, cover with the other plate, flip, and slide the omelette back into the pan, so that the cooked side is on top. Cover and cook for about 5 minutes longer. Cut into wedges and serve.

No Crust Squash-Leek Quiche

This quiche made with squash and leeks is a simple yet elegant main course.

Cook Time: 50 min
Servings: 6

Ingredients

1 large squash

1 Tbsp (15g) butter

2 medium or one large leek, cleaned and chopped

¼ cup (60mL) yogurt

2 eggs

salt

pepper

½ cup (45g) raw cheddar cheese, grated (can be made without

cheese as well)

Directions

Preheat oven to 425F (218 Celsius). Cut the squash in half, scoop out seeds, and then cut the halves into 1-inch (2.5cm) pieces. Place in baking dish with ½ (13mm) an inch of water. Bake until soft, 45-60 minutes.

Meanwhile, roll out pie crust and arrange in pie plate. Poke all over with a fork.

Melt butter, add leeks, and sauté until soft, about 10 minutes.

Beat together eggs, sour cream, salt, and pepper.

When the squash is done, lower oven to 350 (177 Celsius). Transfer squash to the large bowl and mash. Beat in the egg mixture, then stir in leeks.

Spread squash mixture into pie crust and sprinkle with cheese.

Bake until firm and golden, about 45 minutes. When it's nearly done, sprinkle with pine nuts. (They'll burn if they toast for more than a few minutes.)

Remove from oven and let cool for 5 minutes. Slice and serve.

Homemade Mayonnaise

Prep Time: Varies
Makes: 2 cups

Ingredients

1 egg

1 Tbsp (15mL) lemon juice

1 cup (240mL) extra virgin olive oil

2 tsp (10 mL) Dijon mustard

Sea salt and freshly cracked black pepper

Directions

In a blender or food processor, process the egg, lemon juice, mustard, salt and pepper until well combined.

While the motor is running, pour the oil in a slow, thin, steady stream and process until the mixture is thick and creamy

*Take your time with this recipe. If you try and rush it, it won't come out right.

Tangy Egg Salad – No Mayo Recipe

Prep Time: 15 min
Servings: 4-6

Ingredients

2 hard boiled eggs, peeled

2 green onions, finely chopped-green parts only

1 tsp (5mL) worchestershire sauce

1 Tbsp (15mL) Dijon mustard, + more for spreading

1 Tbsp (15mL) lemon juice

Salt and pepper- to taste+plus additional pepper

Directions

Mash eggs together well in a medium sized bowl. I use a fork and/or potato masher.

Add green onions and stir.

Add remaining ingredients and mix well.

Cover and refrigerate overnight.

Mini Vegetable Frittatas

Cook Time: 30-45 min
Makes: 8-10 frittatas

Ingredients

8 large organic eggs

1 Tbsp (15mL) butter

1 cup (120g) zucchini, diced

1 cup (124g) red pepper diced

1 cup (184g) sliced fresh mushrooms

1 leek diced

1 tsp (6g) Celtic Sea Salt

¼ cup (15g) fresh Italian flat leaf parsley, chopped finely

½ tsp (1g) black pepper

½ cup (118 mL) organic milk, preferably raw (I'm going to try and use coconut milk next time and see if that works since I don't eat very much dairy, but I figured I would stick to the recipe exactly as it was written for the first time.)

Directions

Preheat oven to 350 degrees F. Grease a large muffin tin with butter. Whisk eggs and milk together in a large missing bowl. Set aside.

Heat butter in a medium skillet or frying pan over medium heat. Place zucchini, red pepper, mushrooms and leek in a skillet and sauté until vegetables become soft, about 5 minutes. Remove from heat and stir in parsley, salt and pepper. Fold vegetables into egg mixture.

Fill muffin cups three-quarters of the way full with vegetable frittata batter. Bake 20 to 30 minutes until frittatas are set and browned on top.

Serve hot or let cool and store in the fridge for later.

Breakfast Burritos

Cook Time: 5-10 min
Makes: 4 burritos

Ingredients

1-2 Tbsp (5mL) butter

1 small tomato (preferably Roma), chopped

1-2 Tbsp (15-30mL) fresh herbs (thyme, rosemary...), minced

2-3 Tbsp (14-21g) grated raw cheese (optional)

2-3 eggs

2 Tbsp (30mL) soy sauce (wheat free preferably)

¼ cup (30g) chopped walnuts or pecans

½ cup (80g) onion, chopped

Directions

Heat the butter, add onion, and sauté for 3-4 minutes, stirring frequently.

Scramble the eggs.

Add eggs to onions. Cook for 2 minutes; add tomato, soy sauce, and herbs; and heat until warm. Stir in walnuts and optional cheese and remove from stove.

Place half of mixture in a line in the center of each tortilla, leaving 1 inch at either end of the line. Fold each end up to the filling, then fold in one side. Roll. Voilà your breakfast burritos!

Notes   You can leave out the tomato and/or walnuts and/or add other veggies... pretty much whatever you like!

If you don't have any tortillas, you can just serve the filling with some sprouted grain toast or some raw veggies.

Egg Lemon Soup

This interesting, lemony soup is traditional in Greek cuisine. Serve with Greek salad, hummus, and spanakopita for a veggie Greek meal.

Cook Time: 45 min
Makes: 4-6

Ingredients

6 cups (1425mL) vegetable stock

2 egg yolks

1 egg

½ cup (93g) brown rice

¼ cup (59mL) lemon juice

Directions

Bring the stock to a boil, add rice, cover, and cook until tender, 30-40 minutes. You don't need to stir it, but do check on the rice regularly to avoid overcooking.

Just before the rice is done, beat the eggs and yolks until light and fluffy, beat in lemon juice, then beat in 1 cup stock.

Combine the egg lemon with the rice, bring to near boil, stir in parsley, and serve.

Notes: Egg lemon soup is traditionally made with chicken broth, but since lemon is the main flavor, this veggie version tastes almost identical.

Deviled Eggs

Prep Time: 30 min
Makes: 12 halves

Ingredients

6 eggs

2 Tbsp (20g) red onion, minced

1 Tbsp (15mL) soy sauce

1 tsp (5g) dry, yellow, or Dijon mustard

¼ cup (59g) homemade mayonnaise

dash salt

Directions

Place the eggs in the pot and cover with cold water. Once water simmers, cook for 8-10 minutes. Drain the eggs, place in a bowl of cold water, remove one, tap lightly all over until shell cracks, and peel. If it gets too hot to handle, just hold it underwater for a few seconds and try again. (You may need to add more water to the bowl to keep it cold). Peel all of the eggs, then cut in half length-wise. Arrange on a plate.

Pop the yolks out of each half and place in the other bowl, being careful not to break the egg whites. Mash the yolks, then stir in mayonnaise, soy sauce, mustard, onion, and salt.

Take a spoonful of yolk mixture, and use the other spoon to scrape it into one of the egg white holes. Repeat with remaining yolk and whites. If you have some yolk left, just add a bit more to the deviled eggs that don't have enough.

Sprinkle with paprika and/or parsley, and serve.

Deviled eggs are the perfect finger food - you can just grab one and go, so they are great for picnics and parties.

Spanish Tortilla with Zucchini

Cook Time: 1 hour 15 min
Servings: 8

Ingredients

¾ cup (180mL) olive oil

1 large or **3** small zucchini, grated (about 1 pound)

1 lb (450g) potatoes, scrubbed* and diced into ½-inch cubes

1 large onion, chopped

2 tsp (10mL) salt

5-6 eggs

dash of nutmeg

Place grated zucchini in colander, toss with 1 tsp salt, and set in sink or over a bowl to drain.

Heat oil, reduce heat to medium-low, add potatoes, onion, and ½ t salt, and sauté, stirring occasionally, for 30 minutes. If potatoes start to brown, reduce heat.

Squeeze handfuls of zucchini to get rid of as much water as possible, and add the zucchini to the potatoes. Sauté, stirring occasionally, for another 15 minutes. Remove from heat, and use the slotted spoon to transfer vegetables to a large bowl, allowing excess oil to remain in the pan. In the small bowl, beat

Directions

the eggs with remaining ½ tsp salt, nutmeg, and pepper, then stir into the vegetables.

Pour into pan, press everything down lightly, and cook, covered, over very low heat. After 7 minutes, use a rubber spatula to gently lift up one side and check the color of the bottom. When the tortilla is just about set and the bottom is lightly golden (no more than 12 minutes total), remove from heat and let stand, still covered, 5-10 minutes, until set.

Run rubber spatula all the way around the pan to make sure the tortilla isn't stuck anywhere. Place plate upside-down over pan and quickly (and carefully!) flip both, so that the top of the tortilla is now the bottom.

Slide tortilla back into the pan and cook over low heat for another five minutes. Let cool and serve.

No need to peel the potatoes - they are soft and delicious in this tortilla, plus there's lots of nutrients in the skin.

This is a strange recipe in that it's good hot, but it's great at room temperature, so the leftovers are even better than the original dish.

Metabolism Type Test

Adapted from The Metabolic Typing Diet (Wolcott and Fahey 2000, 135), this simple test is the most basic way to determine your metabolism type.

Circle the answer that best completes the following 25 statements according to how you actually feel, not how you think you should feel. If you don't usually pay attention to your body's cues before and after eating, then do so for a few days (while continuing your present eating habits) before taking the test. To ensure a valid result, be honest and do not skip any questions!

Instructions for scoring follow.

Questions

1. When I feel anxious, angry, or irritable,
   A. heavy fatty foods such as meat or salty nuts make me feel better.
   B. fruit, vegetables, or fruit juice makes me feel better.

2. I feel best when I eat the following for breakfast:
   A. sausage, eggs, and/or bacon.
   B. cereal, fruit, and/or toast.

3. If I attended a buffet and could eat whatever I wanted (all health rules aside), I would choose
   A. steak, pork chops, ribs, gravy, and a salad with creamy dressing.
   B. chicken, turkey, fish, vegetables, and a dessert.

4. I feel best when the temperature is
   A. cool or cold; I don't like hot weather.
   B. warm or hot; I don't like cold weather.

5. Coffee makes me feel
   A. jittery, jumpy, nervous, hyper, shaky, or hungry.
   B. okay, as long as I don't drink too much.

6. In the morning, I am
   A. hungry and ready to eat breakfast.
   B. not hungry and don't feel like eating.

7. At midday, I am
   A. hungry and ready to eat lunch.
   B. not noticeably hungry and have to be reminded to eat.

8. In the evening, I am
   A. hungry and ready to eat dinner.
   B. not noticeably hungry and have to be reminded to eat.

9. I concentrate best if I have eaten a meal that includes
   A. meat and fatty foods.
   B. fruits, vegetables, and grains.

10. When I have cravings, I tend to want
   A. salty and fatty snacks (peanuts, cheese, or potato chips).
   B. baked goods or other carbs (bread, cereal, or crackers).

11. When I eat sugar or a sugary snack,
   A. I feel a rush of energy, then am likely to crash and feel fatigued.
   B. my energy levels are restored.

12. If dessert is served,
   A. I can take it or leave it; I would rather have cheese, chips, or popcorn.
   B. I definitely will indulge; I like to have something sweet after a meal.

13. If I have a dessert, I most often choose
   A. cheesecake or creamy French pastries.
   B. cakes, cookies, or candies.

14. For dinner, I feel best (satiated) after eating
   A. steak and vegetables.
   B. skinless chicken breast, rice, and a salad.

15. I sleep best if my dinner is
   A. heavy and includes more proteins.
   B. light and includes more carbohydrates.

16. I wake up feeling well rested if
   A. I don't eat sweets in the evening.
   B. I eat sweets in the evening.

17. I feel best during the day if I eat
   A. small meals frequently, or three meals a day plus some snacks.
   B. two to three meals a day and no snacks; I can last pretty long without eating.

18. I describe myself as someone who
A. loves to eat; food is a central part of my life.
B. is not very concerned with food; I may forget to eat at times.

19. If I skip a meal, I feel
A. irritable, jittery, weak, tired, or depressed.
B. okay; it doesn't really bother me.

20. If I had fruit and low-fat cottage cheese for lunch, I would feel
A. hungry, irritable, and sleepy soon after.
B. satisfied and probably could go until dinner after that.

21. During the day, I feel hungry
A. often and need to eat several times a day.
B. rarely and have a weak appetite.

22. I would describe myself as someone who is more
A. extroverted—I am a very social person.
B. introverted—I usually keep to myself.

23. When a food or meal is very salty,
A. I love it!
B. I don't enjoy it.

24. If I get hungry midafternoon, I feel best (more energized) after eating
A. cheese and nuts.
B. something sweet.

25. After exercising, I feel best if I eat
A. a protein shake or food that contains protein.
B. a high-sugar drink or food, such as a Gatorade or a banana.

Scoring

First, count how many times you circled A and B to determine your scores:

Total number of A answers = _____

Total number of B answers = _____

Next, referring to these scores, select your metabolism type classification according to the following criteria:

- If your A score is 5 or more points higher than your B score (e.g., A = 15, B = 10), then you are a Protein Type.

- If your B score is 5 or more points higher than your A score (e.g., A = 10, B = 15), then you are a Carb Type.

- If your A and B scores are within 3 points of each other (e.g., A = 14, B = 11), then you are a Mixed Type.

This is a copy of the Chapter on Metabolism Types from the Manual for your quick reference. After you have completed the Metabolism Type Test, read through the description of (and special considerations for) your metabolism type in this chapter. You must understand why certain foods are ideal so that you can then make the best choices for your personal meal plan.

As you learn about your metabolism type in this chapter, remember that each person is unique, so some fine-tuning may be necessary as you change your eating habits. Pay close attention to your body's cues. Most people have fallen out of touch with their bodies and don't know what true health feels like. Pay close attention to the one and only source that knows what's best for you—your body!

Protein Types

Protein Types typically crave rich, fatty foods such as pizza, sausages, and salty roasted nuts. If you are a Protein Type, chances are that you love food. You may not feel satiated after a snack and may often feel hungry, even after eating a large meal. When you have eaten too many carbohydrates, you tend to crave sugar. And once you start eating sugary foods, you want more and more and may find it difficult to stop. Sugar often causes you to feel jittery and will quickly make your energy levels drop.

Protein Types may have tried to lose weight by using extreme calorie-cutting methods, only to be unsuccessful—and feel miserable in the process. Protein Types cannot successfully lose weight by drastically decreasing calorie intake.

When Protein Types eat the wrong kind of food, they may notice energy problems—extreme fatigue or a wired "on edge" feeling. Eating often makes them feel better when they feel anxious, nervous, or shaky, but then they feel worse soon afterward. These cycles of energy ups and downs are definite signs of a mismatch between metabolism type and food consumption.

What Does a Protein Type Need?

Protein Types need a diet high in proteins and fats and low in carbohydrates. But think balance—not the Atkins Diet! Protein Types can eat various carbohydrates in the form of some grains, fruits, and vegetables, as long as they are adequately balanced with proteins and fats.

Because Protein Types metabolize food more quickly than other metabolism types (which is why they feel hungry all the time), heavier protein choices such as whole eggs, dark-meat poultry, beef, and dairy are essential for ideal meal planning. These foods have long been considered "unhealthy" because of their high fat content, but as you will learn in the Chapter on Fats, saturated fat is not the cause of disease; refined carbohydrates, processed foods, and hydrogenated oils are. Protein Types who do not eat heavy proteins with a high fat content will be hungry all day and struggle with their weight. Even worse, they will almost always feel fatigued and anxious.

"Must Dos" for Protein Types

- Eat protein at every meal and with every snack. Eating only carbohydrates at a meal causes your blood sugar to spike and then drop quickly, which will leave a Protein Type feeling hungry, fatigued, and anxious as well as cause cravings for more carbohydrates shortly afterward. Eating protein—especially animal protein—at every meal and for snacks will help to control your blood sugar levels and leave you feeling satiated and steady throughout the day. Again, remember to listen to your body; pay attention to which meals and snacks leave you hungry or craving more.

- Eat small meals frequently or healthy snacks between meals. Protein Types need to eat often; otherwise, they'll suffer from extremely low blood sugar levels. Going too long between meals (or snacks) also will create ravenous hunger, which in turn will cause overeating at the next meal—only to lead to lethargy and

- an uncomfortable feeling afterward.

- Avoid refined carbohydrates. Foods such as bread, crackers, and pastas—especially those made from wheat—can be extremely disruptive for Protein Types. Wheat breaks down into sugar faster than any other grain and causes the rapid release of large quantities of insulin. That is why sprouted whole grain bread products are the only allowable sources of bread on the Program. These products are described in the Chapter on Grains.

- Avoid most fruits and fruit juices. Fruits are a wonderful, healthy food, but Protein Types need to be extra careful with their fruit selections. Some fruits are quickly converted to sugar in the bloodstream and cause extreme blood sugar fluctuations. The best fruit choices for Protein Types are apples and avocados (high in fiber and low in sugar). Some people may be able to eat more of these fruits than others.

Carb Types

A Carb Type tends to have a weak appetite. If you are a Carb Type, chances are that you're happy with a minimal amount of food each day. You can get by on small amounts of food and don't give food much thought until you feel hungry.

Carb Types tend to eat less often because they "have no time to eat." These goal-oriented workaholics will skip meals to do what they need to do each day. They may go for extended periods without eating, sending the metabolism into starvation mode. Decreasing the metabolic rate in this fashion can lead to weight management problems and obesity. Carb Types also are more dependent on caffeinated beverages to get them through the day than other metabolism types are. This dependency often weakens their appetites even more, compounding their nutritional problems. Carb Types have a high tolerance for baked goods and starchy vegetables. This can be a bad thing, because they tend to overeat these carbohydrates, which can lead to unhealthy conditions such as hypoglycemia, insulin resistance, and diabetes.

What Does a Carb Type Need?

A Carb Type needs a diet composed of more carbohydrates than proteins or fats. But that doesn't mean that Carb Types don't need protein throughout the day. Lighter, low-fat proteins such as white-meat poultry and whitefish (e.g., tilapia, sea bass) are good choices. Carb Types can choose from a wide variety of carbohydrates and can eat them in larger quantities than any other type.

Although Carb Types convert carbohydrates into energy slowly (unlike Protein Types), it does not mean that they can go on carbohydrate binges. An elevated insulin response is still a concern, especially if weight loss is the goal. Insulin is a fat-storing hormone, so large quantities in the bloodstream will make losing weight quite difficult. Remember, excess of any particular food can lead to weight gain and disease, and always maintain the food portions and ratios recommended for your type (according to the Ideal Food Ratios For Each Metabolism Type Chart).

Carb Types lose weight and feel well on a high-carbohydrate, low-fat diet—the opposite of what a Protein Type needs.

"Must Dos" for Carb Types

- Choose low-fat proteins. Incorporate a low-fat protein such as white-meat poultry or whitefish into each meal. Avoid (or eat only occasionally) high-fat proteins, which may cause lethargy, depression, or fatigue.

- Choose dairy products carefully. Carb Types tend to metabolize dairy poorly. The best way to learn whether dairy is a wise choice for you is to carefully monitor your reaction after you have consumed it with a meal. If you feel lethargic or fatigued shortly after, limit your dairy consumption.

- Choose carbohydrates carefully. Choose plenty of low-starch vegetables, like broccoli and salad greens, and limit consumption of high-starch foods such as bread, pasta, and grains. If you feel sluggish, sleepy, or hungry soon after a meal containing a low-fat protein, a vegetable, and a grain, you may have eaten too much grain. Try increasing the protein amount and decreasing the grain amount the next time you have this same meal.

- Monitor your response to legumes. Carb Types typically cannot easily digest the type of protein that most legumes contain. Therefore, eat legumes infrequently. As with all other foods, monitor your response carefully, and pay attention to your ability to combine them with certain foods. I have some clients who can eat chicken, beans, and vegetables and feel great but feel tired and sluggish if they eat beans, rice, and vegetables.

- Limit the nuts and seeds. Carb Types feel best on a low-fat diet, and nuts and seeds add too much fat to a meal. Nuts and nut butters are great protein choices or snacks, but lean animal meats are better protein choices for meals.

Mixed Types

A Mixed Type requires an equal balance of proteins, carbohydrates, and healthy fats, and including variety in the everyday meal plan is essential. Of the three metabolism types, this one is actually easiest to manage, because the food choices are greater. Some meals may resemble those for Protein Types, and some may resemble those for Carb Types; some may have features of both.

The appetite of a Mixed Type tends to vary greatly throughout the day—hungry at meals but not in between; ravenous at times and no appetite at others. Of course, these responses depend on what foods have been eaten that day. Mixed Types generally don't suffer from cravings. However, like the other types, Mixed Types who eat too much sugar or carbohydrates may develop strong sugar cravings.

Mixed Types must incorporate high-fat and low-fat proteins as well as high-starch and low-starch carbohydrates into their meal plans. If you are a Mixed Type, familiarize yourself with the requirements of both types to find your perfect balance.

A Mixed Type may be more of a Protein Mixed Type or a Carb Mixed Type—in other words, have more qualities of one type than the other. The only way to truly figure this out is by trial and error: by paying close attention to responses to each meal and then determining which foods make you feel good and energized and which foods leave you feeling hungry, fatigued, cranky, or craving more. Finding the right balance of proteins, carbohydrates, and fats is the key to losing weight, feeling great, and achieving optimal health.

The Done For You Meal Plans

By this point you should have read all of Part 1 in The Beyond Diet Manual. If you have also completed Part 2, great! That will be extremely helpful.

Make sure you have completed:

- The Metabolism Typing Test. You should know whether you are a Protein, Carb or Mixed type so you can choose the correct meal plans for you. Remember, if you have any doubt at all about your specific type, you can begin with the Mixed Type meal plans and they will be very effective.

- Your specific calorie calculations and portion requirements. If you haven't done so already, make sure to calculate you calorie requirements in Chapter 4 and then choose the portion requirements that are specific for you from the "Allowable Servings Guide" Sheet.

- The food choices sheet may also come in handy as you use these meal plans to find the best and most appropriate serving sizes for you.

That's all the information you will need to use these delicious meal plans.

Making each meal plan specific for you.

Below you will find meal plans that will make putting together your food for the day a cinch. I will take you through one example so you know exactly how to use each one for your specific needs.

Example:

- A 180 pound person who does moderate weight training

- Calorie Requirements: 2,000 calories per day for weight loss.

- They are a Protein Type.

Using the Allowable Servings Guide, they have found their specific portions for each meal to be:

Breakfast:	3 Protein, 1 Carb
Snack:	3 Protein, 1 Carb
Lunch:	5 Protein, 1 Carb, 2 Fat
Snack:	3 Protein, 1 Carb
Dinner:	5 Protein, 1 Carb, 2 Fat

Using Protein Type Meal Plan #1, this is what their day would look like:

Food		Servings		
Qty	Item	P	C	F
	BREAKFAST			
3 oz	Lamb, Chicken, or Turkey sausage	3		
1 cup	Mushrooms and spinach		1	
	Coconut oil			Use as needed
	SNACK			
1 cup	Sliced celery and carrots		1	
3 Tbsp	Walnut butter	3		
	LUNCH			
5 oz	Beef burger	5		
1 cup	Spinach salad with celery, cauliflower and cucumbers		1	
2 tsps oil	Apple cider vinegar and olive oil			2
	SNACK			
1 small	Green apple		1	
3	Hardboiled eggs	3		
	DINNER			
5 oz	Beef steak	5		
1 cup	Steamed carrots and cauliflower		1	
2 tsps	Butter			2

Remember that this is just a starting point for you to see how your body feels with this quantity of food throughout the day. Some may feel too full, while others may feel hungry and others may feel that it is perfect. It is extremely important that you make notes of those feelings and body cues in your Success Journal. This will help you modify your daily food intake to make it perfect for you.

Please refer to the Allowable Servings Guide and Food Choices table.

Protein Type Meal Plans

Protein Type Meal #1

	Food			
Qty	**Item**	**P**	**C**	**F**
	BREAKFAST			
	Lamb or Pork sausage			
	Mushrooms and spinach			
	Coconut oil			
	SNACK			
	Sliced celery and carrots			
	Walnut butter			
	LUNCH			
	Beef burger			
	Spinach salad with celery, cauliflower and cucumbers			
	Apple cider vinegar and olive oil			
	Raspberries			
	SNACK			
	Green apple			
	Hardboiled eggs			
	DINNER			
	Beef steak			
	Steamed carrots and cauliflower			
	Butter			

Protein Type Meal #2

Food		Servings		
Qty	Item	P	C	F
	BREAKFAST			
	Eggs (poached or scrambled) with Spinach			
	Canadian Bacon			
	Sprouted grain bread or apple			
	SNACK			
	Almonds or walnuts			
	Pear			
	LUNCH			
	Chicken or turkey (dark meat) grilled or baked			
	Carrot Sticks			
	Brown Rice			
	Green Salad w/apple cider vinegar and olive oil			
	SNACK			
	Macadamia Nut butter			
	Celery sticks and Carrot Sticks			
	DINNER			
	Salmon (broiled)			
	Green beans			
	Baked potato			
	Butter			
	Green Salad w/apple cider vinegar and olive oil			

Protein Type Meal Plan #3

Qty	Food / Item	Servings P	C	F
	Food	**Servings**		
Qty	**Item**	**P**	**C**	**F**
	BREAKFAST			
	Pork, Beef or Turkey Bacon			
	Cream of Rice (hot cereal)			
	SNACK			
	Almond or walnut butter			
	Apple			
	LUNCH			
	Shrimp (grilled)			
	Avocado			
	Lentils (cooked)			
	SNACK			
	Raw vegetables with olive oil			
	Sunflower seeds			
	Pear			
	DINNER			
	Beef steak (broiled)			
	Cauliflower (raw or steamed)			
	Brown rice			
	Butter			
	Salad w/apple cider vinegar and olive oil			

Protein Type Meal #4

Food		Servings		
Qty	Item	P	C	F
	BREAKFAST			
	Oatmeal (cooked with water, add cinnamon)			
	Almonds or Walnuts			
	SNACK			
	Blueberries			
	Cashews			
	Pear			
	LUNCH			
	Ground Beef (in a burger or chili)			
	Kidney beans			
	Romaine lettuce and tomato salad			
	Olive oil			
	SNACK			
	Walnut, almond or pecan butter			
	Celery and carrot sticks			
	DINNER			
	Chicken thighs or legs			
	Spinach (sautéed in coconut oil)			
	Couscous			
	Cucumber and tomato salad			
	Apple Cider vinegar and olive oil			

Protein Type Meal #5

Food		Servings		
Qty	**Item**	**P**	**C**	**F**
	BREAKFAST			
	Leftover chicken leg			
	Leftover spinach			
	Apple			
	SNACK			
	Pumpkin Seeds			
	Pear			
	LUNCH			
	Canned Sardines (in olive oil or water)			
	Brown rice			
	Asparagus (steamed)			
	Green salad w/apple cider vinegar			
	SNACK			
	Cashews			
	Carrot sticks			
	DINNER			
	Pork chop (grilled or broiled)			
	Cauliflower (steamed)			
	Butter			
	Quinoa			
	Sliced cucumbers			

Protein Type Meal #6

	Food	Servings		
Qty	Item	P	C	F
	BREAKFAST			
	Eggs (omelet)			
	Peppers, onions and mushrooms			
	SNACK			
	Cashews or cashew butter			
	Banana			
	LUNCH			
	Beef burger			
	Portabella mushroom cap			
	Romaine lettuce, carrot, and celery salad			
	SNACK			
	Apple cider vinegar and olive oil			
	Walnut or Almond butter			
	Celery sticks			
	DINNER			
	Chicken thighs			
	Spinach (sautéed)			
	Spaghetti squash (baked)			
	Butter			

Protein Type Meal #7

Qty	Food Item	Servings P	C	F
	BREAKFAST			
	Chicken sausage			
	Scrambled eggs (or eggs)			
	Butter			
	SNACK			
	Green apple			
	Almond butter			
	LUNCH			
	Chicken legs			
	Romaine salad with celery, carrots and olives			
	Fresh lemon juice and olive oil			
	Blueberries			
	SNACK			
	Pear			
	Pecans			
	DINNER			
	Chicken legs			
	Steamed green beans			
	Butter			
	Blueberries			

Protein Type Meal #8

Qty	Item	P	C	F
	BREAKFAST			
	Bacon			
	Egg omelet with spinach and asparagus			
	Coconut oil			
	SNACK			
	Sardines in olive oil			
	Brown rice crackers			
	LUNCH			
	Baked salmon			
	Spinach salad with beets			
	Apple cider vinegar and olive oil			
	Steamed asparagus with butter			
	SNACK			
	Macadamia nuts			
	Sliced celery			
	DINNER			
	Ocean perch			
	Baked okra and cauliflower			
	Butter			

The table header row: Food (Qty, Item) | Servings (P, C, F)

Protein Type Meal #9

Qty	Food	Servings		
	Item	P	C	F
	BREAKFAST			
	Raw egg shake with ground flax seeds, coconut butter,			
	cream, a banana and cinnamon			
	SNACK			
	Beef burger			
	Carrot sticks			
	LUNCH			
	Spinach salad with chopped celery, avocado, and cucumbers			
	Fresh lemon juice and olive oil			
	Ground dark turkey meat			
	Strawberries			
	SNACK			
	Pumpkin seeds			
	Celery sticks			
	DINNER			
	Seared dark tuna			
	Stir-fried asparagus, cabbage, peas and bok choy			
	Watercress salad			
	Fresh lemon juice and olive oil			

Protein Type Meal #10

Food		Servings		
Qty	Item	P	C	F
	BREAKFAST			
	Smoked wild salmon rolled up with romaine lettuce			
	Peas and corn			
	Butter			
	SNACK			
	Apple			
	Brazil nuts			
	LUNCH			
	Lamb burger			
	Spinach salad with celery, carrots, avocado, artichoke hearts			
	and olives			
	Apple cider vinegar and olive oil			
	SNACK			
	Full fat plain yogurt			
	Blueberries			
	Chopped walnuts and flax oil			
	DINNER			
	Steak			
	Onions sauteed in coconut oil			
	Mixed green salad			
	Apple cider vinegar and olive oil			
	Cherries			

Protein Type Meal #11

Qty	Food	Servings		
	Item	P	C	F
	BREAKFAST			
	Pork sausage			
	Poached eggs			
	Asparagus and mushrooms cooked in butter			
	SNACK			
	Apple			
	Swiss cheese			
	Almonds			
	LUNCH			
	Broiled pork chops			
	Buckwheat grain			
	Steamed green beans			
	Butter			
	SNACK			
	Walnuts or Pecans			
	Celery sticks			
	DINNER			
	Seafood dish: mussels, scallops, squid			
	Quinoa			
	Butter			
	Bibb lettuce salad			

Protein Type Meal #12

Qty	Item	P	C	F
	Food / Servings			
	BREAKFAST			
	Bacon			
	Scrambled eggs			
	Steamed spinach and carrots with butter			
	SNACK			
	Coconut butter			
	Pecans			
	LUNCH			
	Dark meat turkey burger			
	Celery sticks			
	Split pea soup			
	SNACK			
	Carrots and Peppers			
	Hardboiled eggs			
	DINNER			
	Lamb chops			
	Spinach salad			
	Apple cider vinegar and olive oil			
	Steamed beets and cauliflower			
	Butter			

Protein Type Meal #13

Qty	Food	Servings		
	Item	P	C	F
	BREAKFAST			
	Steak			
	Eggs			
	Mashed sweet potato with butter			
	SNACK			
	Celery			
	Peanut butter			
	LUNCH			
	Skirt steak			
	Sugar snap peas			
	Sauteed mushrooms			
	Coconut oil			
	SNACK			
	Coconut butter			
	Pistachios			
	DINNER			
	Roast rack of lamb			
	Steamed asparagus			
	Butter			
	Wild rice			

Protein Type Meal #14

Qty	Food — Item	P	C	F
	BREAKFAST			
	Beef sausage			
	Avocado			
	Olive oil			
	SNACK			
	Carrots and celery sticks			
	Pecan butter			
	LUNCH			
	Beef kidney pate ground with butter, hazelnuts and sea salt			
	Brown rice crackers			
	SNACK			
	Blueberries			
	Coconut butter			
	Raw almonds			
	DINNER			
	Pork chops			
	Steamed cauliflower			
	Olive oil			
	Blueberries			

Protein Type Meal #15

	Food	Servings		
Qty	**Item**	**P**	**C**	**F**
	BREAKFAST			
	Egg omelet with goat cheese and spinach			
	Bacon			
	Coconut oil			
	SNACK			
	Pear			
	Pumpkin seeds			
	LUNCH			
	Ground lamb with spices			
	Butternut squash soup			
	Spinach salad			
	Fresh lemon juice and olive oil			
	SNACK			
	Sliced ham			
	Romaine lettuce			
	Sliced tomatoes			
	DINNER			
	Mackerel with butter and fresh lemon juice			
	Steamed collard greens and beets with butter			

Protein Type Meal #16

Qty	Item	P	C	F
	BREAKFAST			
	Smoked Wild Salmon			
	Tomato slices			
	Avocado and Olive Oil			
	SNACK			
	Cottage Cheese			
	Cucumbers			
	LUNCH			
	Turkey Burger (dark meat)			
	Sprouted Grain bread			
	Lettuce and Tomato			
	SNACK			
	Almond Butter			
	Sliced Apple			
	DINNER			
	Beef shish-ka-bobs			
	Zucchini, red pepper and onion chunks			
	Baked Sweet Potato (sprinkle with cinnamon)			
	Butter (add to potato)			

The header row above the Item/P/C/F row reads **Food** (spanning Qty and Item) and **Servings** (spanning P, C, F).

Protein Type Meal Plan #17

Qty	Food		Servings	
Qty	**Item**	**P**	**C**	**F**
	BREAKFAST			
	Quinoa hot cereal (made with water)			
	Crushed walnuts and pecans			
	(sweeten with stevia or agave syrup and cinnamon)			
	SNACK			
	Hard boiled eggs			
	Raw carrots			
	LUNCH			
	Tuna salad			
	Chopped carrots, celery, and onions (for tuna)			
	Olive Oil			
	Rice Crackers			
	SNACK			
	Greek Yogurt			
	Pumpkin Seeds			
	Strawberries			
	DINNER			
	Venison Stew			
	Carrots, onions and potato (for stew)			
	Raw Cucumber and Celery salad			
	Olive oil			

Protein Type Meal Plan #18

Food		Servings		
Qty	Item	P	C	F
	BREAKFAST			
	Sprouted Grain or Rice Bread			
	Bacon			
	Tomato (Bacon and Tomato Breakfast Sandwich)			
	SNACK			
	Walnuts			
	Cherries			
	LUNCH			
	Venison Stew leftovers			
	Strawberries			
	SNACK			
	Cottage Cheese			
	Blueberries			
	DINNER			
	Duck (baked)			
	Brown Rice			
	Raw Tomato and Onion salad			
	Olive Oil			

Protein Type Meal #19

Qty	Food Item	P	C	F
	BREAKFAST			
	Egg w/ spinach			
	Almond Butter			
	Greek Yogurt			
	SNACK			
	Sliced roast beef roll ups			
	Carrot sticks			
	LUNCH			
	Turkey Chili			
	Kidney beans (for chili)			
	Brown Rice Crackers			
	SNACK			
	Pecans or Pecan butter			
	Banana			
	DINNER			
	Shrimp			
	Coconut Oil			
	Peppers, Onions, Mushrooms (make stir-fry)			
	Wheat free soy sauce			
	Brown Rice			

Protein Type Meal #20

Qty	Food — Item	Servings P	C	F
	BREAKFAST			
	Cottage Cheese			
	Crushed almonds or pecans			
	Blueberries			
	SNACK			
	Hard boiled egg			
	Tomato and cucumber slices			
	LUNCH			
	Chicken drumsticks (baked)			
	Cauliflower (raw or steamed)			
	Butter			
	SNACK			
	Almond butter			
	Celery sticks			
	Apple			
	DINNER			
	Swordfish steak (baked or grilled)			
	Onions (over steak)			
	Corn			
	Green Salad			
	Apple Cider Vinegar and Olive Oil			

Carb Type Meal Plans

Carb Type Meal Plan #1

Qty	Food	Servings		
	Item	P	C	F
	BREAKFAST			
	Chicken sausage			
	Grilled tomatoes, peppers and potatoes			
	SNACK			
	Butter			
	Pineapple chunks			
	Almonds			
	LUNCH			
	Baked flounder			
	Steamed broccoli and beets			
	Mixed green salad			
	Apple cider vinegar and olive oil			
	SNACK			
	Raisins			
	Walnuts			
	DINNER			
	White meat chicken soup with parsley, leeks, peppers,			
	tomatoes, potatoes and onions			

Carb Type Meal Plan #2

Qty	Item	P	C	F
	BREAKFAST			
	Soft-boiled eggs			
	Papaya slices			
	SNACK			
	Sliced turkey breast rolled up with			
	Romaine lettuce			
	Cherries			
	LUNCH			
	White tuna fish			
	Arugula salad with chopped tomatoes, celery, onions, beets			
	and sprouts			
	Fresh lemon juice, olive oil, sea salt and pepper			
	SNACK			
	Full fat yogurt			
	Cucumbers			
	Fresh dill			
	DINNER			
	Baked cod			
	Baked potato with butter			
	Steamed broccoli			

(Food / Servings headers: Food → Qty, Item; Servings → P, C, F)

Carb Type Meal Plan #3

Qty	Food Item	Servings P	C	F
	BREAKFAST			
	Almond or walnut butter			
	Oatmeal (cooked in water, add cinnamon)			
	Strawberries			
	SNACK			
	Cashews			
	Pear			
	LUNCH			
	Ground buffalo (make into chili)			
	Kidney beans (for chili)			
	Sprouted grain bread			
	SNACK			
	Lettuce and tomato salad			
	Peanut butter			
	Celery and carrot sticks			
	DINNER			
	Orange or grapefruit			
	Halibut steak (broiled)			
	Spinach (sautéed)			
	Spaghetti squash (baked)			
	Brown rice			
	Sliced cucumber and tomato salad			

Carb Type Meal Plan #4

Qty	Food Item	Servings P	C	F
	BREAKFAST			
	Scrambled eggs			
	Sprouted grain bread			
	Orange or grapefruit			
	SNACK			
	Almonds or walnuts			
	Apple			
	LUNCH			
	Turkey burger (ground white meat turkey)			
	Brown rice			
	Green salad w/apple cider vinegar and olive oil			
	Pear			
	SNACK			
	Cashew butter			
	Rice crackers			
	DINNER			
	Codfish (baked)			
	Green beans (steamed)			
	Sweet potato (baked)			
	Butter			
	Tomato and cucumber salad w/olive oil			

Carb Type Meal Plan #5

Qty	Food Item	P	C	F
	BREAKFAST			
	Turkey or chicken sausage			
	Cream of rice (hot cereal)			
	Blueberries			
	SNACK			
	Pumpkin or sunflower seeds			
	Banana or apple			
	LUNCH			
	Flounder (broiled)			
	Quinoa			
	Lettuce, tomato, peppers, and cucumber salad			
	Apple cider vinegar and olive oil			
	SNACK			
	Peanut butter			
	Rice crackers			
	DINNER			
	Cornish hen (roasted)			
	Cauliflower (steamed)			
	Sweet potato or yam (baked)			
	Butter			

Carb Type Meal Plan #6

Qty	Food — Item	Servings P	C	F
	BREAKFAST			
	Turkey bacon			
	Millet or quinoa (hot cereal)			
	Grapefruit			
	SNACK			
	Almonds			
	Strawberries			
	LUNCH			
	Chicken (grilled)			
	Kamut (cooked)			
	Lentils			
	Broccoli (steamed or raw)			
	SNACK			
	Walnut butter			
	Celery sticks			
	Grapes			
	DINNER			
	Shrimp or scallops (grilled or baked)			
	Peppers, mushrooms, onions (stir fried)			
	Brown rice			
	Green salad w/apple cider vinegar and olive oil			

Carb Type Meal Plan #7

	Food	Servings		
Qty	Item	P	C	F
	BREAKFAST			
	Hot rice cereal with sunflower seeds, co-conut butter, honey and sliced peaches			
	SNACK			
	Soft-boiled eggs			
	Grapes			
	LUNCH			
	Grilled chicken breast			
	Radicchio and watercress salad with cab-bage, cucumber			
	and leeks dressed in apple cider vinegar and olive oil			
	Baked squash			
	SNACK			
	Peach			
	Almonds			
	DINNER			
	Broiled pork chops			
	Mixed wild and brown rice			
	Romaine salad with peppers, cucumbers and scallions			
	Apple cider vinegar, olive oil, sea salt and pepper			

Carb Type Meal Plan #8

Qty	Food Item	P	C	F
	BREAKFAST			
	Turkey or chicken breakfast sausage			
	Green beans or spaghetti squash			
	Strawberries			
	SNACK			
	Pumpkin seeds			
	Banana			
	LUNCH			
	Mahi mahi (broiled)			
	Romaine, cucumber and tomato salad			
	Apple cider vinegar and olive oil			
	Grapes			
	SNACK			
	Peanut butter			
	Apple			
	Raisins			
	DINNER			
	Cornish hen (baked)			
	Cauliflower (steamed)			
	Broccoli (steamed)			
	Butter			
	Raw red peppers			

Carb Type Meal Plan #9

Qty	Food Item	Servings P	C	F
	BREAKFAST			
	Scrambled eggs			
	Corn polenta			
	Steamed kale			
	SNACK			
	Watermelon			
	Almond butter			
	LUNCH			
	Broiled trout			
	Steamed zucchini and brussels sprouts			
	Butter			
	SNACK			
	Apple			
	Cashew butter			
	DINNER			
	Baked halibut			
	Quinoa			
	Mixed green salad			
	Fresh lemon juice, olive oil, sea salt and pepper			

Carb Type Meal Plan #10

Qty	Food Item	P	C	F
	BREAKFAST			
	Buckwheat pancakes with maple syrup and butter			
	Poached eggs			
	SNACK			
	Sliced tomatoes			
	Turkey Slices			
	LUNCH			
	Chicken or Turkey breast			
	Romaine salad with tomatoes, turnips, zucchini and peppers			
	Apple cider vinegar and olive oil			
	SNACK			
	Strawberries			
	Cottage cheese			
	DINNER			
	Baked tilapia			
	Baked sweet potato			
	Steamed collard greens			
	Butter			

Carb Type Meal Plan #11

Qty	Food Item	P	C	F
	BREAKFAST			
	White tuna salad with chopped apples, cranberries, parsley			
	Celery, honey mustard, olive oil, and sea salt			
	Apple			
	SNACK			
	Steamed brussels sprouts mixed with			
	Pine nuts			
	LUNCH			
	Leftover tuna salad			
	Mixed green salad with cabbage, cucumbers and pine nuts			
	Fresh lemon juice and olive oil			
	SNACK			
	Grapefruit			
	Sliced turkey breast			
	DINNER			
	Broiled trout			
	Brown rice			
	Mixed green salad with sprouts			
	Fresh lemon juice and olive oil			

Carb Type Meal Plan #12

	Food	Servings		
Qty	Item	P	C	F
	BREAKFAST			
	Shake with full fat yogurt			
	Banana and honey			
	Almonds and flax oil			
	SNACK			
	Egg salad with celery, parsley, olive oil, sea salt and pepper			
	Broccoli			
	LUNCH			
	Chicken sausage kabobs			
	Peppers, zucchini, onions			
	Butternut squash soup			
	SNACK			
	Sunflower seeds			
	Cantaloup and honeydew			
	DINNER			
	Halibut			
	Lentils			
	Brown rice			
	Grilled onions			
	Coconut oil			

Carb Type Meal Plan #13

Qty	Food Item	Servings P	C	F
	BREAKFAST			
	Egg omelet			
	Broccoli, onions, tomatoes			
	Coconut oil			
	SNACK			
	Fresh green vegetable juice			
	Almond and Coconut butter (mixed)			
	LUNCH			
	Ground white meat chicken			
	Basmati rice			
	Romaine salad with mixed peppers			
	SNACK			
	Apple cider vinegar and olive oil			
	Mango			
	Sunflower seeds			
	DINNER			
	Baked Cornish hen			
	Steamed beets, cabbage and zucchini			
	Butter			

Carb Type Meal Plan #14

Qty	Food Item	P	C	F
	BREAKFAST			
	Turkey bacon			
	Poached eggs			
	Grapefruit			
	SNACK			
	Sliced cucumber			
	Sliced pepper			
	Almonds			
	LUNCH			
	Cobb salad with romaine, cilantro, turkey breast, hardboiled			
	egg, tomatoes, onions and radishes			
	Apple cider vinegar and olive oil			
	sea salt and pepper			
	SNACK			
	Watermelon			
	Almonds			
	DINNER			
	Fresh water perch			
	Grilled eggplant and garlic			
	Millet grain			
	Olive oil			

Carb Type Meal Plan #15

Qty	Food Item	P	C	F
	BREAKFAST			
	Chicken or Turkey sausage			
	Broccoli			
	Coconut oil			
	SNACK			
	Orange			
	Soft-boiled eggs			
	LUNCH			
	Ground white meat turkey			
	Buckwheat grain			
	Arugula salad with onions, zucchini and peppers			
	Fresh lemon juice and olive oil			
	SNACK			
	Nectarine			
	Almonds			
	DINNER			
	Chicken breast			
	Sweet potato			
	Steamed broccoli			
	Butter			

Carb Type Meal Plan #16

	Food	Servings		
Qty	Item	P	C	F
	BREAKFAST			
	Egg			
	Sprouted Grain or Rice Bread (egg sandwich or French toast)			
	Apple or Apple Sauce			
	SNACK			
	Greek Yogurt			
	Raspberries or Blueberries			
	LUNCH			
	Turkey Breast (sliced)			
	Lettuce and tomato			
	Sprouted Grain, Rice or Spelt Bread			
	Mango slices			
	SNACK			
	Pecans			
	Raisins			
	DINNER			
	Mahi Mahi (grilled or baked)			
	Corn			
	Lettuce, tomato, cucumber, peppers, onion salad			
	Apple Cider Vinegar and Olive oil			
	Cherries			

Carb Type Meal Plan #17

	Food	Servings		
Qty	Item	P	C	F
	BREAKFAST			
	Quinoa hot cereal (made with water)			
	Crushed walnuts and pecans			
	Strawberries			
	SNACK			
	Cottage Cheese			
	Pineapple chunks			
	LUNCH			
	Tuna salad (light tuna)			
	Chopped carrots, celery, and onions (for tuna)			
	Olive Oil			
	Rice Crackers			
	SNACK			
	Yogurt			
	Almonds			
	DINNER			
	Buffalo meatballs			
	Tomato sauce			
	Spelt or Rice Pasta			
	Green salad			
	Apple Cider Vinegar and Olive Oil			

Carb Type Meal Plan #18

	Food	Servings		
Qty	**Item**	**P**	**C**	**F**
	BREAKFAST			
	Veggie Omelet			
	Peppers, onion, tomato, mushrooms			
	Sprouted grain or rice bread			
	SNACK			
	Cashew or Peanut Butter			
	Apple or Pear			
	LUNCH			
	Turkey Burger (light meat)			
	Sprouted Grain bread			
	Lettuce and Tomato			
	Strawberries			
	SNACK			
	Peach			
	Walnuts			
	DINNER			
	Shrimp			
	Coconut Oil			
	Peppers, Onions, Mushrooms (make stir-fry)			
	Wheat free soy sauce			
	Brown Rice			

Carb Type Meal Plan #19

Qty	Food Item	Servings P	C	F
	BREAKFAST			
	Greek Yogurt			
	Strawberries, Blueberries			
	Oatmeal (made with water)			
	SNACK			
	Soft boiled egg			
	Sliced Green, Red and Yellow Peppers			
	LUNCH			
	Shrimp			
	Avocado			
	Tomato and Cucumber salad			
	Apple Cider Vinegar and Olive Oil			
	SNACK			
	Turkey breast slices			
	Rice Crackers			
	DINNER			
	Chicken shish-ka-bobs			
	Zucchini, red pepper and onion chunks			
	Baked Sweet Potato (sprinkle with cinnamon)			
	Butter (add to potato)			

Carb Type Meal Plan #20

Qty	Food / Item	P	C	F
	BREAKFAST			
	Cottage Cheese			
	Crushed almonds or pecans			
	Pineapple chunks			
	SNACK			
	Almond Butter			
	Apple Sauce			
	LUNCH			
	Chicken breast (grilled or baked)			
	Baked Sweet Potato			
	Broccoli (steamed)			
	Butter (for potato and broccoli)			
	SNACK			
	Yogurt			
	Pumpkin seeds and sunflower seeds			
	DINNER			
	Turkey Chili			
	Kidney beans (for chili)			
	Sprouted grain or Spelt tortilla			
	Sliced tomato			

Mixed Type Meal Plans

Mixed Type Meal Plan #1

Qty	Food Item	Servings P	C	F
	BREAKFAST			
	Beef or Pork bacon			
	Grapefruit			
	SNACK			
	Macadamia nuts			
	Celery and carrot sticks			
	LUNCH			
	Chicken breast			
	Steamed broccoli			
	Brown rice			
	Butter			
	SNACK			
	Apple			
	Sliced turkey breast			
	DINNER			
	Lamb chops			
	Chopped tomato, cucumber and onion salad			
	Apple cider vinegar and olive oil			
	Brown rice			

Mixed Type Meal Plan #2

Qty	Food Item	Servings P	C	F
	BREAKFAST			
	Eggs (omelet)			
	Spinach, peppers, and onions (in omelet)			
	Sprouted grain bread			
	SNACK			
	Almonds or walnuts			
	Apple			
	Cucumber slices			
	LUNCH			
	Turkey burger (ground white and dark meat)			
	Carrot sticks			
	Brown rice			
	Sliced tomato			
	SNACK			
	Peanut butter			
	Rice crackers			
	Celery sticks			
	DINNER			
	Halibut steak (broiled)			
	Green beans (sautéed in butter and garlic)			
	Sweet potato (baked)			
	Green salad w/apple cider vinegar and olive oil			

Mixed Type Meal Plan #3

Qty	Item	P	C	F
	Food	**Servings**		
	BREAKFAST			
	Turkey or chicken breakfast sausage			
	Cream of rice (hot cereal)			
	Blueberries or strawberries			
	SNACK			
	Almond or walnut butter			
	Banana or apple			
	Carrot sticks			
	LUNCH			
	Salmon filet (broiled)			
	Sweet potato or Yam			
	Lettuce, tomato, pepper and cucumber salad			
	Apple cider vinegar and olive oil			
	SNACK			
	Pumpkin seeds			
	Pear			
	DINNER			
	Shrimp (stir fried)			
	Peppers, onions, mushrooms (stir fried)			
	Brown rice			
	Sliced cucumbers and carrots			

Mixed Type Meal Plan #4

	Food		Servings		
Qty	Item		P	C	F
	BREAKFAST				
	Scrambled eggs				
	Hot rice cereal (sweetened with stevia or agave syrup)				
	Butter				
	SNACK				
	Celery sticks				
	Almond butter				
	LUNCH				
	Baked salmon				
	Arugula salad with peppers and onions				
	Fresh lemon juice and olive oil				
	Steamed zucchini with butter				
	SNACK				
	Shake with coconut water, pineapple and coconut butter				
	DINNER				
	Flounder				
	Steamed asparagus with butter				
	Sliced avocado				
	Apple cider vinegar and olive oil				

Mixed Type Meal Plan #5

Qty	Food Item	Servings P	C	F
	BREAKFAST			
	Bacon			
	Scrambled eggs			
	Onions sauteed in coconut oil			
	SNACK			
	Banana			
	Almond butter			
	LUNCH			
	Baked Cornish hen			
	Quinoa			
	Spinach and garlic			
	Coconut oil			
	SNACK			
	Sliced turkey breast			
	Romaine lettuce			
	DINNER			
	Broiled pork chops			
	Mixed brown and wild rice			
	Sliced cucumber and tomato			

Mixed Type Meal Plan #6

	Food		Servings		
Qty	Item		P	C	F
	BREAKFAST				
	Egg omelet with mozzarella cheese				
	Tomatoes, mushrooms and onions				
	SNACK				
	Sardines in olive oil				
	Brown rice crackers				
	LUNCH				
	Chicken breast				
	Romaine salad with cauliflower, cucumbers, and celery				
	Fresh lemon juice and olive oil				
	Quinoa				
	SNACK				
	Sliced tomatoes				
	Sliced turkey breast				
	Olive oil				
	DINNER				
	Lamb steak				
	Mixed green salad with broccoli, cabbage and carrots				
	Fresh lemon juice and olive oil				

Mixed Type Meal Plan #7

Qty	Food Item	P	C	F
	BREAKFAST			
	Lamb sausage			
	Steamed kale			
	Corn polenta			
	SNACK			
	Honeydew and Cantaloupe			
	Brazil nuts			
	LUNCH			
	Buffalo burger			
	Mixed green salad with chopped tomatoes and onions			
	Apple cider vinegar and olive oil			
	Steamed brussels sprouts with butter			
	SNACK			
	Sunflower seeds or Pecans			
	Strawberries			
	DINNER			
	Baked cod			
	Steamed cauliflower and turnips			
	Butter			
	Millet			

Mixed Type Meal Plan #8

Qty	Food Item	P	C	F
	BREAKFAST			
	Greek yogurt			
	Blueberries			
	Chopped walnuts and ground flax seeds			
	SNACK			
	Papaya			
	Cashews			
	LUNCH			
	Beef burger			
	Steamed kale and zucchini			
	Olive oil			
	SNACK			
	Baked apples			
	Walnuts			
	DINNER			
	Red snapper			
	Steamed asparagus			
	Sliced avocado			
	Fresh lemon juice and olive oil			

Mixed Type Meal Plan #9

Qty	Food				
	Item	**P**	**C**	**F**
	BREAKFAST			
	Egg (poached or scrambled)			
	Turkey or beef bacon			
	SNACK			
	Oatmeal (cooked with water, add cinnamon)			
	Cashews			
	Pear			
	Celery sticks			
	LUNCH			
	Buffalo (ground and made into chili)			
	Kidney beans (for chili)			
	Lettuce and tomato salad			
	Olive oil			
	SNACK			
	Walnut or pecan butter			
	Celery and carrot sticks			
	DINNER			
	Lean steak (grilled)			
	Spinach (sautéed)			
	Spaghetti squash (baked)			
	Wild rice			

Mixed Type Meal Plan #10

Qty	Food Item	P	C	F
	BREAKFAST			
	Leftover grilled steak			
	Leftover spinach and spaghetti squash			
	SNACK			
	Red apple			
	Pecans			
	Strawberries			
	Sliced cucumbers			
	LUNCH			
	Flounder (broiled)			
	Quinoa			
	Celery, tomato and pepper salad w/ olive oil			
	Butter			
	SNACK			
	Almonds			
	Banana			
	DINNER			
	Cornish hen (baked)			
	Sweet potato (baked)			
	Butter			
	Green salad w/apple cider vinegar and olive oil			

Mixed Type Meal Plan #11

Qty	Food Item	Servings P	C	F
	BREAKFAST			
	Turkey sausage			
	Grilled tomatoes, peppers and onions			
	Potatoes			
	SNACK			
	Almonds			
	Sliced mixed peppers			
	LUNCH			
	Cobb salad with turkey, ham, bacon, eggs			
	Romaine lettuce with carrots and celery			
	Apple cider vinegar and olive oil			
	SNACK			
	Plum			
	Peanuts			
	DINNER			
	Beef chili with onions and tomatoes			
	Red beans			
	Brown rice			
	Mixed green salad			
	Apple cider vinegar and olive oil			

Mixed Type Meal Plan #12

Qty	Food Item	Servings P	C	F
	BREAKFAST			
	White tuna salad with olive oil and honey mustard			
	Chopped apples, cranberries, celery			
	Celery sticks			
	SNACK			
	Apple			
	Pecans			
	LUNCH			
	Lamb burger			
	Steamed swiss chard with butter and garlic			
	Onions sauteed in coconut oil			
	SNACK			
	Carrot sticks			
	Peanut butter			
	DINNER			
	Mahi Mahi			
	Spinach salad			
	Fresh lemon juice and olive oil			
	Buttered corn and carrots			

Mixed Type Meal Plan #13

Qty	Food	Servings		
	Item	P	C	F
	BREAKFAST			
	Poached eggs			
	Feta cheese and spinach sauteed in coconut oil			
	SNACK			
	Carrot and celery sticks			
	Pumpkin seeds			
	LUNCH			
	Mackerel seasoned with butter, fresh lemon juice, parsley,			
	Sea salt and pepper			
	Arugula salad with apple cider vinegar and olive oil			
	Sauteed leeks			
	SNACK			
	Kiwi			
	Macadamia nuts			
	DINNER			
	Baked cornish hen			
	Lentils			
	Basmati rice			
	Cucumber slices			

Mixed Type Meal Plan #14

Qty	Food	Servings		
	Item	P	C	F
	BREAKFAST			
	Turkey bacon			
	Scrambled eggs			
	Watermelon			
	SNACK			
	Apple sauce			
	Peanut butter or almond butter			
	LUNCH			
	Chicken legs			
	Grilled eggplant and garlic			
	Romaine salad with chopped cucumbers and tomatoes			
	Fresh lemon juice and olive oil			
	SNACK			
	Green apple			
	Soft-boiled eggs			
	Sliced tomatoes			
	DINNER			
	Shrimp stir-fry			
	Brown rice			
	Eggs			
	Bok choy, bamboo shoots, eggplant, peppers, and zucchini			

Mixed Type Meal Plan #15

Qty	Food / Item	P	C	F
	BREAKFAST			
	Peanut butter or almond butter			
	Oatmeal (cooked in water, add cinnamon)			
	Blueberries or raisins			
	SNACK			
	Peach			
	Cashews			
	LUNCH			
	Sardines or Salmon			
	Avocado			
	Sliced tomato			
	Olive oil			
	SNACK			
	Sliced turkey			
	Carrots			
	Strawberries			
	DINNER			
	Lamb chop (grilled)			
	Zucchini (green and yellow, grilled)			
	Yam (baked)			
	Butter			

Mixed Type Meal Plan #16

	Food		Servings		
Qty	Item		P	C	F
	BREAKFAST				
	Smoked Wild Salmon				
	Tomato slices				
	Avocado and Olive Oil				
	SNACK				
	Pecan butter				
	Apple				
	LUNCH				
	Turkey Breast (sliced)				
	Lettuce and tomato				
	Sprouted Grain, Rice or Spelt Bread				
	Orange or grapefruit				
	SNACK				
	Greek Yogurt				
	Blueberries				
	DINNER				
	Buffalo meatloaf (used ground buffalo instead of beef in recipe)				
	Sautéed spinach				
	Green salad				
	Apple Cider Vinegar and Olive Oil				

Mixed Type Meal Plan #17

Qty	Food Item	Servings
		P	**C**	**F**
	BREAKFAST			
	Eggs			
	Sprouted grain, Rice or Spelt Bread (egg sandwich or French toast)			
	Orange or grapefruit			
	SNACK			
	Almonds and Pumpkin Seeds			
	Dried Cranberries (no sugar added)			
	LUNCH			
	Chicken breast (grilled or baked)			
	Baked Sweet Potato			
	Broccoli (steamed)			
	Butter (for potato and broccoli)			
	SNACK			
	Cottage Cheese			
	Apple Sauce			
	DINNER			
	Grilled Red Snapper			
	Green beans sauteed with almonds			
	Wild Rice			

Mixed Type Meal Plan #18

Qty	Food Item	Servings P	C	F
	BREAKFAST			
	Quinoa hot cereal (made with water)			
	Crushed walnuts and pecans			
	Raisins or Berries			
	SNACK			
	Soft Boiled Eggs			
	Carrot Sticks			
	LUNCH			
	Turkey Chili			
	Kidney beans (for chili)			
	Sprouted grain or Spelt tortilla			
	SNACK			
	Sliced tomato			
	Peanut butter			
	Raisins			
	Sprouted Grain, Rice or Spelt Bread			
	DINNER			
	Shrimp			
	Coconut Oil			
	Peppers, Onions, Mushrooms (make stir-fry)			
	Wheat free soy sauce			
	Brown Rice			

Mixed Type Meal Plan #19

Qty	Food			
	Item	Servings		
		P	C	F
	BREAKFAST			
	Greek Yogurt			
	Almonds			
	Banana			
	SNACK			
	Turkey breast slices			
	Sliced tomato			
	LUNCH			
	Tuna salad (light or dark tuna)			
	Chopped carrots, celery, and onions (for tuna)			
	Olive Oil			
	Rice Crackers			
	SNACK			
	Cottage Cheese			
	Mango			
	DINNER			
	Lamb burgers			
	Portabella Mushroom Caps			
	Lettuce and tomato			
	Cherries			

Mixed Type Meal Plan #20

Qty	Food Item	Servings P	C	F
	BREAKFAST			
	Beef or Turkey Bacon			
	Sprouted Grain, Rice or Spelt Bread			
	Sliced Tomato			
	SNACK			
	Cashew butter			
	Banana			
	LUNCH			
	Wild Smoked Salmon			
	Avocado			
	Sliced Tomato and Cucumbers			
	SNACK			
	Greek Yogurt			
	Sunflower seeds			
	Blueberries			
	DINNER			
	Buffalo or Beef Chili			
	Kidney beans (for chili)			
	Sprouted grain or Spelt tortilla			
	Sliced tomato			

So...Just Who Is Isabel De Los Rios?

Isabel De Los Rios is a certified nutritionist and exercise specialist

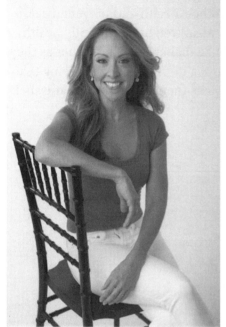

who has already helped more than 300,000 people all over the world lose incredible amounts of weight, regain their health and permanently change their lives. She is the author of The Beyond Diet Program and has become the #1 "go-to girl" when it comes to fat-burning nutrition by several of the most popular fitness professionals around the globe. Isabel's cutting-edge and completely different approach to nutrition is what sets her apart from all the rest. Her strategies work, hands down, as long as her simple principles are followed.

Isabel found her passion for nutrition as a teenager. The overweight daughter and granddaughter of type 2 diabetics, Isabel was told she was doomed to suffer from the same health problems as the generations who preceded her. Not willing to sit around waiting for this grim prediction to become a reality, she pored over every nutrition and diet book available in search of the answers to her family's weight and health problems. This led her to personally seek out doctors and health professionals that were using nutrition to get great results (as far as health and weight loss) with their patients and clients.

Isabel is able to educate clients and readers all over the world through her books, hundreds of online articles, seminars, and the media, focusing on the essential principles of fat-loss nutrition and achieving a healthy, toned, and vibrant body.

Isabel graduated from Rutgers University with a degree in exercise physiology (a pre-med curriculum). She is a Certified Strength and

Conditioning Specialist, the highest and most advanced certification given by the National Strength and Conditioning Association. She is also a Holistic Nutrition Lifestyle Coach, certified by the Corrective Holistic Exercise Kinesiology (C.H.E.K.) Institute in San Diego, California. She counsels many special populations, including people with diabetes and heart disease, cancer survivors, and overweight individuals, as well as healthy individuals who wish to maintain their health and prevent disease. She has since reached and maintained an ideal weight, is vibrantly healthy, and shows no indication that conditions like diabetes will affect her as they have so many in her family. She truly enjoys a high level of well-being that not only surprises most people, but motivates them to achieve what Isabel has.

References

Batmanghelidj, F. (1992). *Your Body's Many Cries for Water.* Vienna, VA: Global Health Solutions, Inc.

Byrnes, Stephen (2001). *The Lazy Person's Whole Foods Cookbook.* Ecclesia Life Man.

Chek, Paul (2004). *How to Eat, Move and Be Healthy.* San Diego, CA: C.H.E.K. Institute.

Daniel, Kaayla T. (2005). *The Whole Soy Story: The Dark Side of America's Favorite Health Food.* Washington, DC: New Trends.

Fallon, Sally, with Mary G. Enig (2001). *Nourishing Traditions: The Cookbook that Challenges Politically Correct Nutrition and the Diet Dictocrats,* 2nd edition. Washington, DC: New Trends.

Fife, Bruce (2001). *The Healing Miracles of Coconut Oil.* Colorado Springs, CO: Health Wise.

Finger Lakes Gourmet (no date). Online recipes. www.fingerlakesgourmet.com, accessed January 2007.

Free-Gourmet-Recipes.com (no date). Healthy Recipes. www.free-gourmet-recipes.com, accessed June 2008.

Kirsch, David (2005). *The Ultimate New York Body Plan.* New York, NY: McGraw-Hill.

Lanctôt, Guylaine (1995). *The Medical Mafia: How to Get Out of It Alive and Take Back Our Health and Wealth.* Morgan, VT: Here's The Key Inc.

Mercola, Joseph (2005). *Dr. Mercola's Total Health Program: The Proven Plan to Prevent Disease and Premature Aging, Optimize Weight, and Live Longer.* Schaumburg, IL: Joseph Mercola. Available from www.mercola.com/forms/total_health_book.htm, accessed June 2008.

Mercola, Joseph (no date). *The Truth About Coconut Oil: Why It Got a Bad Rep.* articles.mercola.com/sites/articles/ archive/2003/09/13/coconut-oil-part-three.aspx, accessed June 2008.

Mercola, Joseph, with Rachael Droege (2003). *Trans Fat: What Exactly Is It and Why Is It So Dangerous?* www.mercola.com/2003/ jul/19/trans_fat.htm, accessed June 2008.

Mercola, Joseph, with Alison Rose Levy (2003). *The No-Grain Diet: Conquer Carbohydrate Addiction and Stay Slim for the Rest of Your Life.* New York, NY: Dutton. Available from www.mercola.com/ nograindiet, accessed June 2008.

Quillin, Patrick (2005). *Beating Cancer With Nutrition.* Carlsbad, CA: Nutrition Times Press.

Regenerative Nutrition (no date). *Celtic Ocean Sea Salt.* www. regenerativenutrition.com/content.asp?id=30, accessed June 2008.

Rubin, Jordan S. (2004). *The Maker's Diet.* Lake Mary, FL: Siloam.

Sears, Al (no date). Dr. Sears Made a Mistake ... *Doctor House Call* 78. www.alsearsmd.com/content/index.php?id=doctor_house_ call_78&no_cache=1&sword_list[]=Coconut&sword_list[]=Oil, accessed June 2008.

Simopoulos, Artemis P., and Jo Robinson (1998). *The Omega Diet: The Lifesaving Nutritional Program Based on the Diet of the Island of Crete.* New York, NY: Harper Collins.

Wild Oats Marketplace (no date). *Online Recipes.* www.wildoats. com, accessed January 2007. (Editor's note: Wild Oats is now Whole Foods Market. Visit the Whole Foods Recipe Index: www. wholefoodsmarket.com/recipes/index.html, accessed June 2008.)

Wolcott, William, and Trish Fahey (2000). *The Metabolic Typing Diet.* New York, NY: Doubleday.

NOTES:

NOTES:

www.BeyondDiet.com